African Medicine

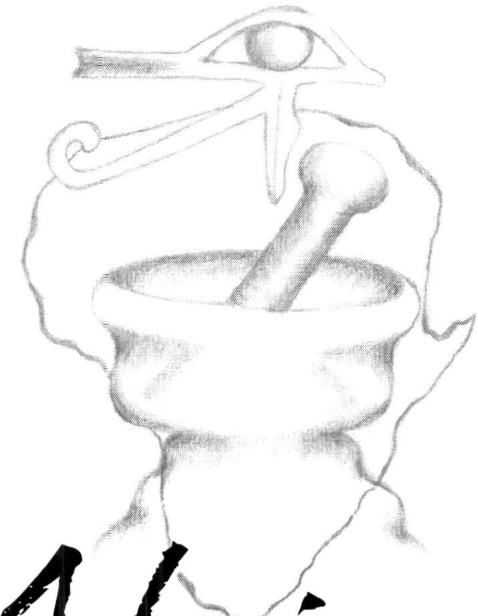

African Medicine

A SPIRIT SCIENCE OUT OF THE SHADOWS

Charles S. Finch III, M.D.

First Publications of Finch Essays
"The African Background to Medical Science" in *Journal of African Civilizations*, Vol. 4, No. 1, 1982, New Brunswick, NJ, Journal of African Civilizations Ltd., Inc.

"Imhotep the Physician: Archetype of the Great Man" in *Great Black Leaders: Ancient and Modern*, Ivan Van Sertima, editor, New Brunswick, NJ: Journal of African Civilizations Ltd., Inc., 1988.

"Science and Symbol in Egyptian Medicine: Commentaries on the Edwin Smith Papyrus" in *Egypt Revisited*, 2nd edition, Ivan Van Sertima, editor, New Brunswick, NJ: Journal of African Civilizations Ltd, Inc., 1989.

Second Publication
Finch, Charles S. *The African Background to Medical Science: Essays on African History, Science & Civilizations*. United Kingdom: Karnak House, 1990.

Author photo: Kemit P. Finch
Cover artwork: Camille Nixon Johnson
Cover design: Deb Tremper, Six Penny Graphics

ISBN: 978-0-9629444-5-1

Library of Congress Control Number: 2025906704

Printed in the United States of America by BCP Digital Printing.

Contents

Acknowledgements

I first acknowledge Ivan Van Sertima, who encouraged me to research and write my first article, *The African Background to Medical Science*. He then printed my articles in his *Journal of African Civilizations*, thus launching my writing and speaking career. Van Sertima subsequently gave permission for these articles to be published by Karnak House (*The African Background to Medical Science: Essays on African History, Science, and Civilizations*. United Kingdom: Karnak House, 1990). I will always be grateful to Amon Saba Sakana for the opportunity he gave me to present to a wider audience a compilation of all the essays I had written in the 1980's.

Some 43 years later, with Karnak House relinquishing its publication rights to Khenti, Inc., I have compiled the original articles about medicine in Africa into this single book. *African Medicine: A Spirit Science Out of the Shadows* could not have come into being without the expertise of Deb Tremper of *Six Penny Graphics* who painstakingly reformatted every page in Chapters 3, 5, and 6 from my only copy of the original Karnak House book. She also reviewed each photo and illustration, bringing out the best in every one. I give thanks to my wife, Ellen Finch, for revising and updating the original articles, as well as for guiding and managing the business aspects of the book's publication. Dr. Toni Briegel created the index, which is so important in an educational text.

I wish to thank Jewel L. Crawford, M.D. for referring me to the article described in Chapter 3 by ReFaey et. al. (2019) that links the Eye of Horus to the brain's sensory system. This book includes information on traditional medicine in Africa. My insights on this subject were enhanced through my experiences in Senegal, West Africa under the leadership of Maam Fatou Seck and her Ndeppkats who allowed me to participate in spiritual ceremonies and witness healings. I am also thankful to USAID for a grant which allowed me to investigate the medical practices of the Saltigues of Malango. Erick Gbodossou, M.D., founder of the Experimental Center for Traditional Medicine at Malango and President of *PROMETRA* International, provided important insights into the philosophy and practices of traditional African healers. Virginia Davis Floyd, M.D., MPH provided valuable updates on the work of *PROMETRA* International, including information on the partnership of the organization with the Morehouse School of Medicine that led to the research on HIV/AIDS. Iris Green and Lenny Foster, master photographers, and Dr. Virginia Floyd contributed numerous photos to this work. Invaluable technical and marketing expertise was provided by Frank Lewis. Finally, I thank the late Dr. Mwalimu Imara of the Morehouse School of Medicine for encouraging me to compose the *Oath of Sunu* in 1985.

I give the highest praise to African medical practitioners, both male and female, who over thousands of years, have cared for and continue to provide healthcare to their people in body, mind, and spirit without any of today's modern medical technology.

Charles S. Finch III, M.D.
March 9, 2025

Introduction

It has been customary to think that the formal discipline of medical science in the modern sense is not, nor has ever been, intrinsic to Africa. Africa is supposedly a land bereft of any science or advanced knowledge. This is "cognitive dissonance" of an extraordinary degree. Clearly, as is so often the case in the historical relations between Europe and Africa, the reality is one thing, the propaganda another. Most of the work in this genre has been encumbered with assumptions about the primacy of Greece—and by contradistinction, the utter deficiency of Africa—in the evolution of medical science. It is as if such pre-ordained ideas were so intrinsically correct that they required no proof or demonstration.

The beginnings of the healing profession are lost in the dim mists of prehistoric antiquity. Healing as a vocation can be said to have begun at the time when a remote, nameless human ancestor—taking cues from the habits of animals—brought leaves, grasses or roots to an ill relative in an attempt to relieve his distress. The origin and evolution of healing as a special skill long antedates other important human inventions such as agriculture and animal domestication and might well deserve consideration as "the oldest profession." The accumulated observations and trials of thousands of years brought a wealth of healing knowledge to mankind, and by the historical era, medicine as a systematic discipline, as a veritable science, had emerged—in Africa.[1]

As with so many other human achievements, a formal medical science emerged first in the Nile Valley, reaching its highest level of development—until modern times—in Egypt, land of the pharaohs. When Egyptian dynastic history begins, medicine is already an established, fully-formed science. This we know from the most important medical text-books of ancient Egypt, now known as the Ebers Papyrus and the Edwin Smith Papyrus, which are in fact copies of medical papyri which date back to pre-pyramid times, to the very earliest historical dynasties. In point of fact, one of the pharoahs of the 1st dynasty was famous as a physician.[2] From the beginning of her history, Egypt possesses a mature, well-validated system of medicine containing a systematic pathology, a completely-formulated pharmacopeia, a formal knowledge of anatomy and physiology, a large medical literature, a well-defined medical teaching curriculum, and a skill in surgery and trauma that is hardly matched outside Africa until our own time.

It is unthinkable that such knowledge, which is so sophisticated on a scientific level, could have emerged without a long period of anterior development. There is a 2400-year span from Hippocrates to modern medicine, and the mature medical

1 See Finch, C. *Echoes of the Old Darkland: Themes from the African Eden*, 1991, Decatur, GA, Khenti, Inc., pp. 1–51, for a discussion of the beginnings of mankind in Africa.

2 According to Manetho, the second pharaoh of the 1st dynasty, Athothis, son of Menes, was a great physician who wrote treatises on anatomy. It is therefore just possible that this personage had a hand in writing the treatise that in a much later redaction became the Edwin Smith Papyrus. By the "short chronology" this would put the original of the Edwin Smith Papyrus back to 3000 B.C.; by the "long chronology" back to 4000 B.C. All this furnishes additional evidence showing that Egyptian medicine was already a mature science at the very beginning of Egyptian dynastic history.

science that exists at the start of the dynastic period in Egypt would have had a pedigree at least as long. If we date the onset of Egyptian dynastic history around the first *known* calendar date of 4236 B.C., which the author believes is closer to the actual beginnings of Egyptian dynastic history rather than the conventional 3200 B.C., our best educated guess would push the origins of Egyptian medicine back, close to 7000 B.C., and very possibly much earlier. There is a persistent emphasis in most writings about Egyptian medicine on its "static" quality, which is to say the priest/physicians of ancient Egypt followed ancient, pre-established authority so rigidly that they were incapable of any scientific innovation or evolution in this domain. On the face of it, such a conclusion is tenuous at best, and in any case does not account for how the Egyptians got to such an advanced stage in the first place. If Egyptian medicine was of a caliber beyond that of all later medicine up to our own time, we have to presume that not only was the scientific spirit alive and well in ancient Egypt, but that it actually originated there.

Is ancient Egypt separate from the rest of Africa? Egypt itself grew out of much older civilizations in Africa.[3] Research by African historians shows that groups migrated over a period of time out of the Nile Valley to the west and south, and that they brought their culture with them to be passed on through their carefully preserved oral teachings. It is now evident that Africans all over the continent are closely related through mythology, religion, culture, language that can be traced back to Egypt and

3 Finch, C., *Nile Valley Civilization: A 10,000-year History*, 2021, Ellenwood, GA, Khenti, Inc.

the Nile Valley.[4] Why is this fact important? Conventional historians have a respect and admiration for ancient Egyptian culture and religion that does not extend to the rest of Africa. In this work, the author invites us to look for deeper meaning in African traditional religion, medicine, and science, and to celebrate the genius that has survived for thousands of years in all parts of Africa through wars, enslavement, and colonialism.

It must be noted that when we speak of African physicians, we are really describing African physician/priests, a concept very different from the medical doctors we are familiar with in the West who are primarily medical scientists. "Science is a recent method of looking at things," says J. Olumide Lucas.[5] Historically, the roles of physician and priest were deeply intertwined across various cultures. What we now think of as "magic" was part of the training and craft.[6] A healing procedure might require medicines, but also incantations, prayers, information from dreams and/or divinations, and sacrifice. Even the inappropriate and derogatory term, "witch-doctor," used to incorrectly describe African medical practitioners in years past, suggests a blending of the spiritual/magical/occult realm with physical methods. African healing interventions operate on multiple levels—biophysical, psychic, energetic, spiritual, and cosmic—interacting seamlessly within a multidimensional model of the human self and an energetic connection with all of nature.

4 Lucas, J.O., *The Religion of the Yorubas*, 1996, Brooklyn, NY, Athelia Henrietta Press, Inc., pp.18–30 Also in Diop, C.A. Precolonial Black Africa, 1987, Brooklyn, NY, Lawrence Hill Books, pp.215–216.

5 op. cit., Lucas p.341

6 Brier, B. *Ancient Egyptian Magic,* 1980, New York, William Morrow and Company, Inc., Bob Brier, p.34

The essence of human consciousness and its development has been intricately tied to the concept and practices surrounding sacrifice. This phenomenon is not only a central theme in mytho-religious contexts globally but has a special resonance within African spiritual systems, where it is seen as an innate component of the life process itself. Since the inception of life some 12 billion years ago, existence is perceived as a continuous journey of becoming. This transformative process is manifested in various forms, with "beingness" as a constant amidst change, perpetually undergoing organization, disorganization, and reorganization. The intricate relationship between life and death is such that each element defines and enables the other, creating a complex interplay essential for the evolution of existence. This dynamic is further highlighted by the African philosophical view that life and death are not opposing forces, but complementary elements in a continuous dance.

Throughout history, African people have learned to use plants as medicine. Herbal medicine in Africa is thousands of years old. All over the continent, native peoples developed an extensive pharmacopeia, revealing a thoroughly empirical and rational knowledge of the medicinal applications of hundreds of plants. We are beginning to realize that with the demise of the ancient knowledge, was a loss of techniques that modern science has not yet discovered, acknowledged, invented, or recovered. To this end, the author has included as an appendix to his research a Knowledge, Attitudes, and Practices (KAP) study on traditional healers in Fatick, Senegal, who may be among the last of their kind.[7] The most critical issue

7 Finch, Charles, *A Knowledge, Attitudes, and Practices Survey of Traditional Healers in Fatick, Senegal;* this survey was funded by a grant from the United States Aid to International Development #685-0281-G-00-1254-00, 199

facing the world in the next millennium is how to live on the earth without destroying it. Increasingly, we are beginning to suspect that the ancients, in Africa (and elsewhere) had, in fact, solved this problem. Their buried knowledge may hold the key to the future for everyone.

This book only scratches the surface of a topic as old as humanity itself. Future exploration into African medicine will rely on a collective, global reconciliation to the fact that civilization, like the human race itself, began in Africa.

Charles S. Finch, III, M.D.

CHAPTER ONE

The African Background of Medical Science

Summary: It has become increasingly clear that traditional African cultures and civilizations knew and accomplished much more than has traditionally been assumed. Even after we've "restored" ancient Egypt—a civilization that was the fountainhead of science—to its true and natural place on African soil as an African creation, there is yet a profound reluctance to admit that Africa contributed anything of substance to world science.

Just as any discussion of the achievements of Western medicine harkens back to Hippocrates and Galen, so any discussion of African medical achievements harkens back to ancient Egypt. Newsome, among others, has shown what a debt Greek medicine owed to the priest-physicians of Egypt.[1] Not only was the most important Greek healing deity, Asclepios, identified with the legendary Egyptian physician—architect-aphorist Imhotep—but Hippocratic therapeutics had direct antecedents in Egyptian medicine. The city-state of Athens used to import Egyptian physicians, as did most of the kingdoms of the Near East, and in the

1 Newsome, F: "Black Contributions to the Early History of Western Medicine", *Journal of African Civilizations,* 2(1&2): 27–39, 9/80.

Odyssey, Homer says, "In medical knowledge, Egypt leaves the rest of the world behind".[2]

Like all African medicine, Egyptian medicine has baffled scholars because of the complete interpenetration of "magico-spiritual" and "rational" elements. Mostly, this magico-spiritual aspect has been downplayed or belittled. However, at least one researcher concedes that healing, being a complicated psychic as well as physical process, may be amenable to an approach that touches that hidden area of the psyche beyond the reach of rational therapy.[3] Even modern medicine concedes that as much as 60% of illness has a psychic base and indeed, the well-known "placebo" effect of modern pharmaco-medicine arises from this.[4] We moderns like to deride this magico-spiritual medicine but it can and does produce startling results that we do not understand.

The Egyptians were writing medical textbooks as early as 5,000 years ago.[5] This indicates not only a mature civilization but also a period of medical development. Out of the hundreds and thousands of medical papyri that must have been written, only 10 have come down to us, the most important being the Ebers and Edwin Smith Papyri. These 10 papyri form the basis of most of what Egyptologists know about Egyptian medicine. It has been affirmed, however, that much of the training and instruction

2 Quoted in Sigerist, H. *E.,A History of Medicine: Primitive and Archaic Medicine.* New York, Oxford University Press, 1951, p. 325.

3 Ghalioungui, P., *The House of Life: Magic and Medical Science in Ancient Egypt.* Amsterdam, BM Israel, 1973.

4 A placebo is a pharmacologically inactive drug which the patient believes is active. In many illnesses, the mere act of believing in the efficacy of the medicine can give beneficial results in 40% or more of patients. Without this effect, faith healers would have gone out of business centuries ago. An interesting recent article is "The Placebo Effect" in the April, 1981 issue of *MD* magazine.

5 Sigerist, op. cit., p. 300.

of the healing priests must have been orally transmitted, as it is in the rest of Africa.[6] It is likely, therefore, that we have only a partial grasp of the true scope of Egyptian medical knowledge. Moreover, like their counterparts in the rest of Africa, the Egyptian priest-physicians often kept their best knowledge secret.

Egyptian physicians were instructed in the "per ankh" or "house of life" which served as a university, library, medical school, clinic, temple, and seminary. The numerous Greek philosophers who studied in Egypt, such as Pythagorous, Thales, and Plato, must have spent their time in a *per ankh.* In these centers of learning, there was no sharp demarcation between the fields of study. Religion, philosophy, science, astronomy, mathematics, music, and hieroglyphics were all part of the same species of knowledge and were reflected in one another.

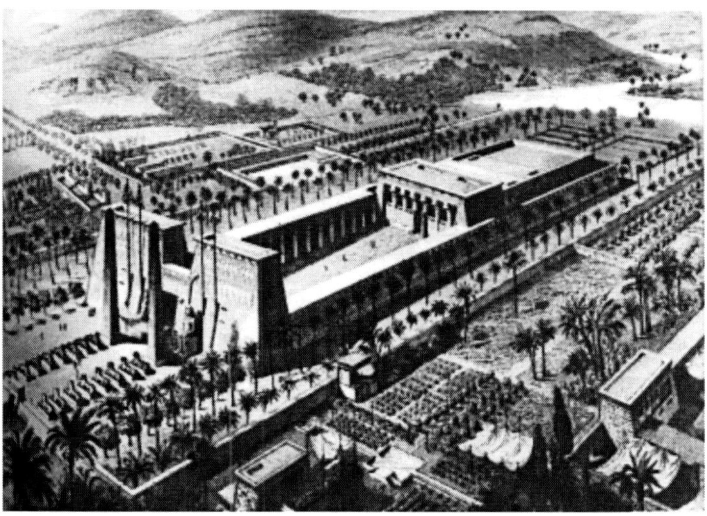

Figure 1
EGYPTIAN PER ANKH (House of Life) *EDFU TEMPLE*

6 Ghalioungui, op. cit., p. 30.

It is of interest that the Egyptians were alone among the nations of antiquity in the development of specialty medicine. In the Old Kingdom, the diseases of each organ were under the care of a specialist. In the later epochs, the specialists disappeared as the Egyptian physician began to function as a generalist. However, during Ptolemaic times, specialization came back into vogue, probably as a result of renewed interest in the archaic culture. Not until the 20th century did anything comparable in the sphere of medicine develop. Contemporary doctors are accustomed to believing that modern specialty medicine resulted from a progressive evolution of medical techniques and knowledge, hardly realizing that it is a throwback to the earliest form of Egyptian medical practice.

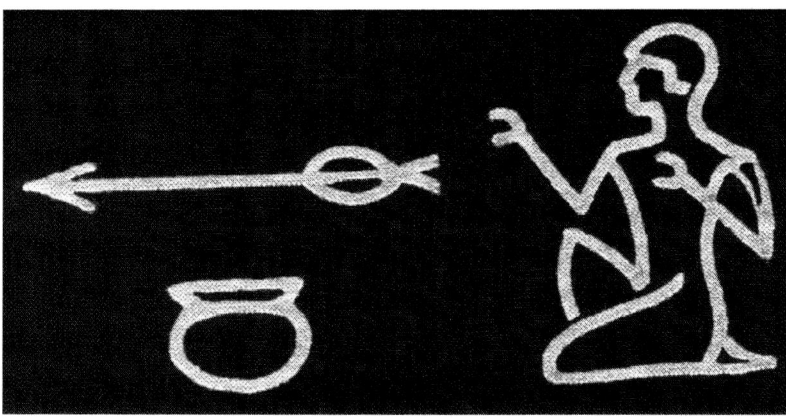

Figure 2
SUNU (sūnū)
The Physician of Ancient Egypt

A study of ancient Egyptian diagnostic methods reads disconcertingly like a modern textbook on physical diagnosis. A physician summoned to examine a patient would begin with a careful appraisal of the patient's general appearance. This would be followed by a series of questions to elicit a description of the complaint. The colour of the face and eyes, the quality of nasal secretions, the presence of perspiration, the stiffness of the limbs or abdomen, and the condition of the skin were all carefully noted. The physician was also at pains to take cognizance of the smell of the body, sweat, breath, and wounds. The urine and feces were inspected, the pulse palpated and measured, and the abdomen, swellings, and wounds probed and palpated. The pulse-taking is worth noting because it indicates that the Egyptians knew of its circulatory and hemodynamic significance. Percussion of the abdomen and chest was performed and certain functional tests we still use today were done, i.e., the coughing test for hernia detection; the extension-flexion maneuver of the legs to test for a dislocated lumbar vertebra. Sometimes, the case required more than one consultation and the physician might, as is done today, embark on a "therapeutic trial" to ascertain the efficacy of treatment. It also seems that the Egyptians practised a form of socialized medicine. All physicians were employees of the state and medical care was available to everyone.[7]

The extant medical papyri show us that the Egypians had quite an extensive knowledge of anatomy and physiology. They understood the importance of pulsation and—4500 years before Harvey—knew something of the structure and function of the cardiovascular system. They knew that the heart was the centre of this system, had names for all the major vessels, knew the relation between heart and lung, and knew the distribution of the vessels through the limbs.[8] They had names for the brain and

7 Sigerist, op. cit., p. 323.
8 Ghalioungui, op. cit., pp. 49, 51.

meninges (the covering of the brain and spinal cord) and also seem to have known the relation between the nervous system and voluntary movements. In addition, the ureters (the connections between the kidneys and the bladder) were known and named. Most writers state that the Egyptians' anatomical knowledge, while relatively sophisticated, was, by modern standards, rudimentary. They aver, for example, that the Egyptians attached no special significance to the brain.[9] But at least one researcher, utilizing sources entirely different from the papyri, contradicts this notion, asserting that their knowledge of neuro-anatomy in particular was as detailed and advanced as that in modern times.[10]

The Egyptians were well-versed in many pathological syndromes. The identification of a disease necessitates acute and painstaking clinical observation, often over many years, and many of the ones described in the medical papyri are known today. Egyptian physicians understood the origin of paraplegia and paralysis from spinal cord injuries and recognized the traumatic origin of neurological symptoms such as deafness, urinary incontinence, and priapism. They described many syndromes of cardiac origin. They knew that excess blood in the heart and lungs was pathological which is consistent with what we know about congestive heart failure today. They also seem to have recognized the significance of heart palpitations and arrhythmias and gave a rather precise definition of angina pectoris:

9 Reeves, C, "Illustrations of Medicine in Ancient Egypt", *J. Audiov Media Med,* 3(1), 5, 1/80.

10 Schwaller de Lubicz, R. A., *The Temple in Man,* trans. D. Lawlor, Brookline, Autumn Press, 1977.

> If thou examinest a man for illness in his cardia and he has pains in his arms, in his breast, and on one side of his cardia... it is death threatening him.[11]

The modern description of angina pectoris can hardly improve upon this. The phrase seen in the Ebers Papyrus, "belly too narrow for food", seems to indicate an esophageal or stomach stricture perhaps from an inflammatory or ulcerating process. Egyptian physicians also knew that a weak heart adversely affected the liver, calling to mind the pathological enlargement of the liver which we know to be due to heart failure. Faintness due to a "dumb heart" was described which seems to be an allusion to a Stokes-Adams attack.[12] It is evident that the ancient Egyptian physicians had a fundamental grasp of the pathophysiology of many of the syndromes we know today.

Perhaps the most remarkable document among the medical papyri is the surgical Edwin Smith Papyrus, a compendium of Egyptian anatomical knowledge and surgical methods. It is in this papyrus that the remarkable descriptions of the traumatic surgical lesions and their treatment are found. We also find that the priest-physicians also recognized the signs and symptoms of sciatica, the sharp pain radiating down the leg caused by nerve compression in the lower spinal cord. Like many other peoples in Africa and the rest of the world, the Egyptians practiced trephi-

11 Ghalioungui, op. cit., p. 123.

12 A modern medical textbook says this about Stokes-Adams attacks: "Syncopal (fainting) attacks... are common in Type II block, and they have the characteristics of all such syncopal attacks that are due to a *sudden cessation of circulation.*" (emphasis mine) *Harrison's Principles of Internal Medicine,* Thorn, Adams, et al, editors, New York, McGraw Hill, 1977, p. 1203. Compare this to an inscription in the Ebers Papyrus: "as to faintness: it is that the heart does not speak or that vessels of the heart are dumb..." Ghalioungui, op. cit., p. 217.

nation.[13] This operation, the forerunner of neurosurgery, involves boring a hole through the skull to the outer covering of the brain. This was done to remove fragments from a skull fracture compressing the brain, to treat epilepsy, or to relieve chronic headache. Today in Africa there are people who have undergone this operation with no apparent ill effects and there are skulls from ancient Egyptian graves with definite signs of healing around the trephination site, so it is clear that patients have survived this operation.

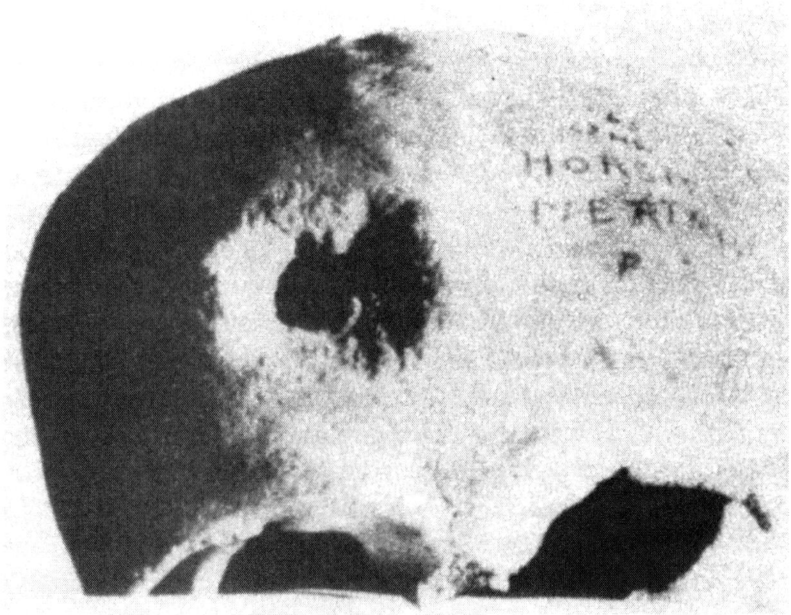

Figure 3

Skull with frontal hole, a trephine hole or a healed skull wound. Museum of Anatomy, Cairo Faculty of Medicine.

13 Ghalioungui, op. cit., p. 89.

As is seen very commonly in Africa, there was a separate guild of bonesetters in Egypt who treated fractures and dislocations. These specialists devised a completely effective method for reducing collar bone fracture which Hippocrates later used.[14] The Edwin Smith Papyrus also describes maneuvers for reducing dislocated jaws and shoulders. Long bone fractures were immobilized with tight splints and nasal fractures were treated by the insertion of stiff nasal packings into the affected nostril, a method also used today for uncomplicated nasal fractures.

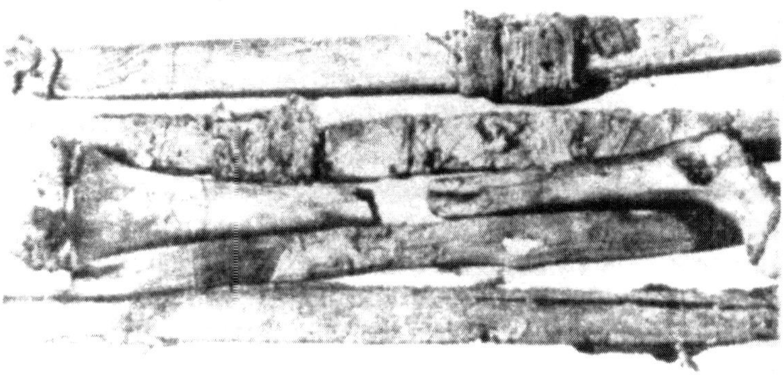

Figure 4
Splints of wood padded with vegetable fibre, surrounding a broken femur. Cairo Faculty of Medicine.

The Egyptians had perhaps three to four thousand years of experience dissecting and bandaging mummies and this must have had beneficial effects on surgical technique. They had an array of knives and scalpels to excise tumours and drain abscesses. They used red-hot metal instruments to seal off bleeding points and closed clean wounds with sutures or adhesive tape. They were unsurpassed as bandagists and used their techniques to control

14 Ibid., p. 42.

bleeding. Fresh meat was also used to stop oozing hemorrhage from surgical wounds. Like the ancient Chinese, they used molds from bread or cereals to treat wound infections. Modern penicillin was extracted from a mold so the priest-physicians must also have been aware of its bacteriacidal properties.

Like all African peoples, the Egyptians had a large *materia medica,* using as many as 1000 animal, plant, and mineral products in the treatment of illness. The Egyptians extracted oils from plants and trees and used them as perfumes and medicines (these are some of the same 'essential oils' we know and use today). Night blindness, caused by vitamin A deficiency, was treated with ox livers, known to be rich in vitamin A. Poppy extract—the source of opium-was used to treat colicky babies. Modern physicians use paregoric—whose active ingredient is opium—for exactly the same purpose. Patients with scurvy—caused by vitamin C deficiency—were fed onions, a known source of vitamin C. This is the first example of vitamin therapy in the world. The ancient physicians of the Nile Valley recognized that metabolic imbalances caused by nutritional deficiencies caused disease.

Castor seeds, the source of castor oil, were used to make cathartic preparations. Mandrake and henbane, sources of belladonna alkaloids, were also known and used. The belladonna possess properties that stimulate the heart, decrease stomach motility, dilate the pupils, and cause sedation. Honey was used in ⅓ part to ⅔ parts of grease as a wound salve. It has been reliably demonstrated that such a concoction hastens wound healing and reduces infection, even in modern surgical theatres.[15] The Egyptians dis-

15 Rosenthal, Elizabeth, *4,000 Year-old treatment revived to heal wounds,* New York Times, April 5, 1990.

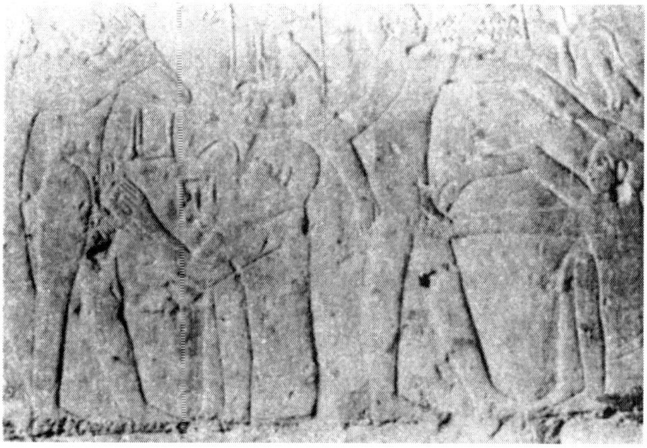

Figure 5a

Circumcision: Tomb of Ankh-ma-Hor (Sesi) in Saqqara. Right: the surgeon rubs on something with an ovoid instrument. The patient says: "Rub well the part". Answers the operator: "I shall make it so that it is so agreeable". Left: the cutting. Operator to assistant: "Hold him well, do not let him fall down". Assistant: "I shall do what you praise me for".

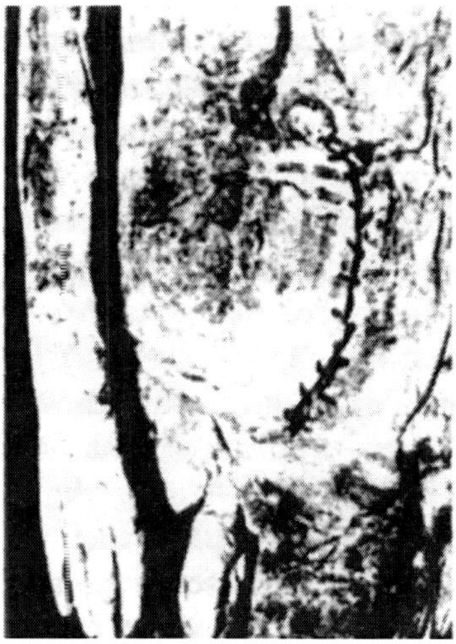

Figure 5b

Gaping wounds were probably stitched as seen at right on a mummy's abdomen.

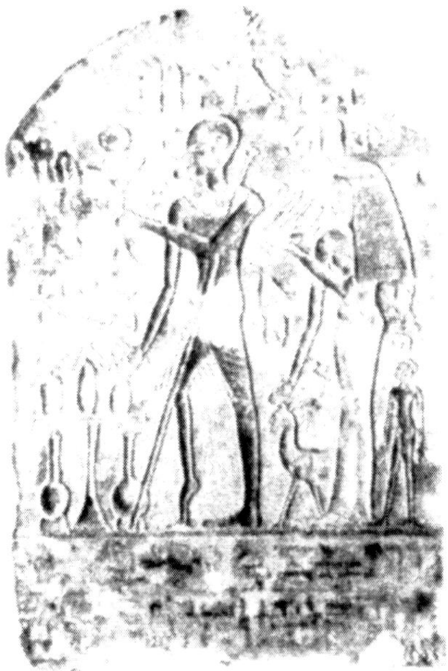

Figure 6
A mandrake root being offered to Akhenaten by his wife Nefertiti.

pensed their prescriptions as pills, enemas, suppositories, infusions, and elixirs in accurate, standardized doses, causing some to wonder if they had separate pharmacies and pharmacists.[16]

Most of us are familiar with the story of gold, frankincense, and myrrh being presented as gifts to the Christ child. When cuts are made in the bark of different species of Commiphora (myrrh) and from the Boswellia (frankincense) trees, a sap containing natural fungicides and bactericides oozes out and hardens into a resin which can be scrapped off. The Egyptians commonly used frankincense and myrrh antimicrobial resins in mumification, as incense and perfumes, and in treating wounds and skin sores. Myrrh, in particular was used to treat pain, inflammatory condi-

16 Ghalioungui, op. cit., pp. 148–9.

tions, sore throats, diarrhea, and periodontal diseases (gingivitis). The scents of frankincense and myrrh are said to have a mood elevating, but relaxing and calming effect that facilitates meditation. These resins were considered sacred and were burned as incense in Egypt from antiquity. There is a famous story of Queen Hatshepsut sending a voyage to Punt to obtain myrrh trees.

Today, frankincense and myrrh are popular homeopathic remedies throughout the world. Current studies have focused on applying clinical trial methodologies to validate the use of myrrh as an antineoplastic, an antiparasitic agent, and as an adjunct in healing wounds.[17] In another study, myrrh from *Commiphora molmol* was found to kill bacteria without the bacteria becoming resistant to it.[18]

Egyptian art often shows men and women wearing cosmetics, especially around the eyes. In earlier periods of Egyptian history, green malachite was crushed into a powder to create this "make-up." The green color was thought to offer spiritual protection, but was found also to prevent inflammation of the eyes.[19]

17 El Ashry, El-Sayed H, Rashed, N, Salama, O M, Saleh, A. "Components, Therapeutic Value and Uses of Myrrh," *Pharmazie* 58: 163–168 (2003), Alexandria University, Ibrahimia, Egypt

Also Nomicos EY. Myrrh: medical marvel or myth of the Magi? Holist Nurs Pract. 2007 Nov-Dec;21(6):308-23. doi: 10.1097/01.HNP.0000298616.32846.34. PMID: 17978635.

Also Schwarcz J, "A Myrrhy Christmas." Mcgill OSS Weekly Digest, 18 Dec 2018, Mcgill Office of Science and Society.

18 Bhattacharjee MK, Alenezi T. Antibiotic in myrrh from *Commiphora molmol* preferentially kills nongrowing bacteria. Future Sci OA. 2020 Feb 20;6(4):FSO458. doi: 10.2144/fsoa-2019-B

19 Metwaly AM, Ghoneim MM, Eissa IH, Elsehemy IA, Mostafa AE, Hegazy MM, Afifi WM, Dou D. Traditional ancient Egyptian medicine: A review. Saudi J Biol Sci. 2021 Oct;28(10):5823-5832. doi: 10.1016/j.sjbs.2021.06.044. Epub 2021 Jun 19. PMID: 34588897; PMCID: PMC8459052.

Later in Egyptian history, kohl was used, which consisted of a mixture of crushed galena (a mineral found in the mountain regions of Sinai), and lead. Lead, however, is known to be toxic to humans. Tapsoba, et. al. (2010) found in examining Egyptian make-up samples from the Louvre, that lead was used "sparingly" in the composition of the make-up. In this limited amount, the lead actually boosted production of nitric oxide in human cells.[20] Nitric oxide is a molecule synthesized in our bodies which boosts our immune defenses. "The present data thus establish that the eyes of Egyptians bearing the black makeup were presumably prone to immediately resist a sudden bacterial contamination with extreme efficiency through the spontaneous action of their own immune cells."[21] Eye infections caused by dust and flies were especially common during periods when the Nile flooded creating marshy areas with stagnant water which

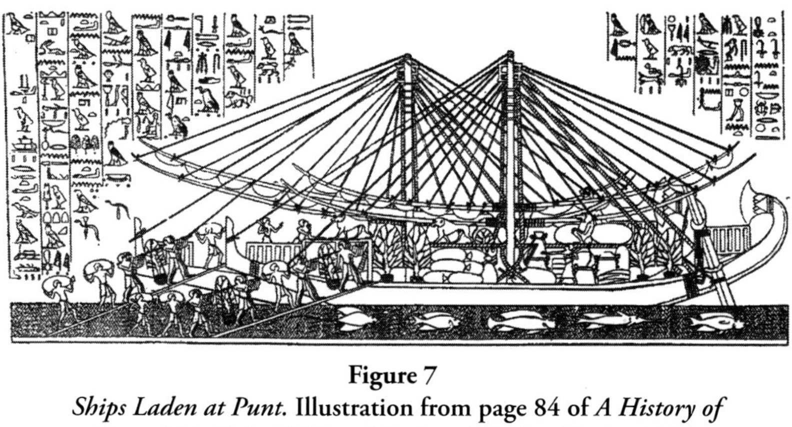

Figure 7
***Ships Laden at Punt.* Illustration from page 84 of *A History of Egypt*, Vol. II, by William Matthew Flinders Petrie, 1896.**

20 Tapsoba I, Arbault S, Walter P, Amatore C, "Finding Out Egyptian Gods' Secret Using Analytical Chemistry: Biomedical Properties of Egyptian Black Makeup Revealed by Amperometry at Single Cells." *Analytical Chemistry* 2010 *82* (2), 457–460. DOI: 10.1021/ac90234

21 Ibid.

became contaminated.[22] The eye paint also protected eyes from the sun's glare (football players today smear a dark powder around their eyes for the same reason).

The Egyptians were fastidious about personal hygiene. They bathed their bodies in the morning, before meals, and in the evening, and of course, bathed their feet in special foot basins. They even used body deodorants, toothpaste, and breath mints, to keep themselves fresh.

Breath mints: frankincense, cinnamon, melon, pine seeds, and cashews were mixed together, and ground into a powder. Honey was added. The honey mixture was heated over a fire, left to cool slightly, and then formed into small candies.[23]

Deodorant: "A recipe and prescription from the medical text known as the Hearst Papyrus recommends mixing lettuce, myrrh, incense, and another plant (whose name is not known), and rubbing the paste on the body to prevent the odor of perspiration. The juices from fruits, mixed with frankincense or other spices, such as cinnamon, were also used."[24]

Toothpaste was made from rock salt, mint, dried iris flower and grains of pepper, which were crushed and mixed together. The mixture was then moistened with one's own saliva, and sticks, fashioned into crude "toothbrushes," were also used.[25] The toothpaste was reconstituted at a dental conference in Vienna in 2003. One dentist who attended the meeting commented: "Nobody in

22 Ibid.

23 Mark, J. J. (2017, May 04). *Cosmetics, Perfume, & Hygiene in Ancient Egypt. World History Encyclopedia.* Retrieved from https://www.worldhistory.org/article/1061/cosmetics-perfume--hygiene-in-ancient-egypt/

24 Ibid.

25 Ibid.

the dental profession had any idea that such an advanced toothpaste formula of this antiquity existed."[26]

Several goddesses were patron deities of medicine and healing. All physician-priests of ancient Egypt, for example, were priests of the goddess Sekhmet, the lion-headed goddess who, among other things, brought famine, pestilence, and death. She presided as the goddess of physicians because she could prevent or ward off such life-threatening disasters as well as bring them on. The ancient hippopotamus goddess Ta-Urt presided over child birth. She was often represented as a hippopotamus standing on her hind legs, huge belly protruding in the fashion of pregnancy, cupping a breast as if she is getting ready to suckle an infant. Isis, particularly in the latter phases of Egyptian history, became a pre-eminent goddess of healing through the phenomenon of 'incubation.' A sick patient would be brought to her temple and given a sleeping draught. Isis would then come to the afflicted person in a dream and instruct him/her what to do in order to be healed.

Women were physician-priestesses who often wielded significant ecclesiastical power. The goddesses, of course, each had their own colleges of priestesses but from about 1,570 BC on, there was always in place a Chief Prophetess or Divine Adoratrice of Amon, a position usually held by the Great Royal Wife. Amon was the supreme deity of ancient Egypt from 2,200 BC to 120 BC so the Chief Prophetess of Amon was very much like a female pope.

The Egyptians were also quite knowledgeable in handling obstetric and gynecological problems. They knew and treated uterine prolapse. They had means of inducing abortions and preventing

26 Zoech, Irene, The ancient Egyptian recipe for toothpaste, *The Telegraph*, 19 January 20

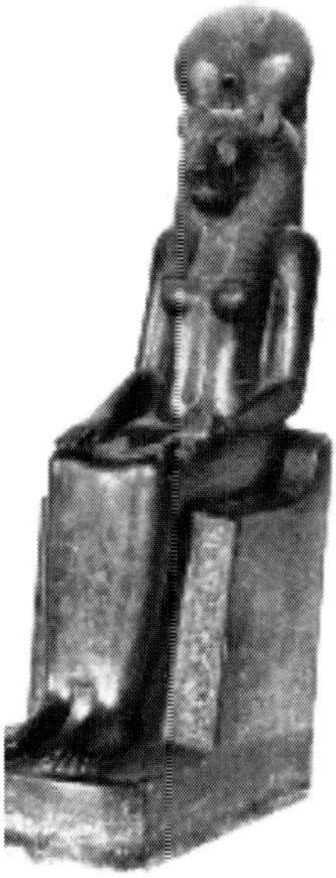

Figure 8
SEKHMET:
Goddess of Physicians

conception. They even had an effective pregnancy test! A sample of a woman's urine was sprinkled on growing cereals; if the cereals did not grow the woman was considered not pregnant; if they did grow she was declared pregnant. Modern experiments have shown that a pregnant woman's urine has a permissive effect on the growth of barley in about 40% of the cases, demonstrating that there must have been some validity in the world's first pregnancy test.[27]

There are nearly 120 physicians listed in Egyptian annals; four of them are women. The most important of these was Peseshet of the Middle Kingdom, who was not only a trained physician, but was, in the course of her career, promoted to chief of physicians.[28]

27 Ibid., pp. 112–3.
28 Ghalioungui, Paul, *The Physicians of Pharaonic Egypt, National Library of Medicine*, 1983, p.18, p.92. Ghalioungui assumes that Peseshet is a chief of women physicians particularly instead of physicians generally.

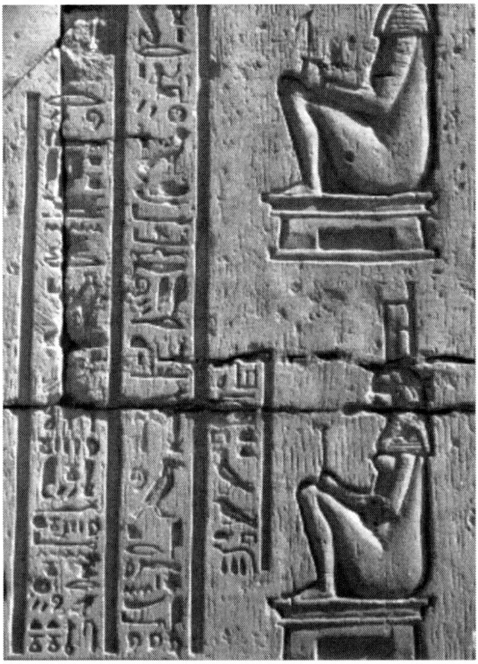

Figure 9
Ancient Egyptian Birthing Chair

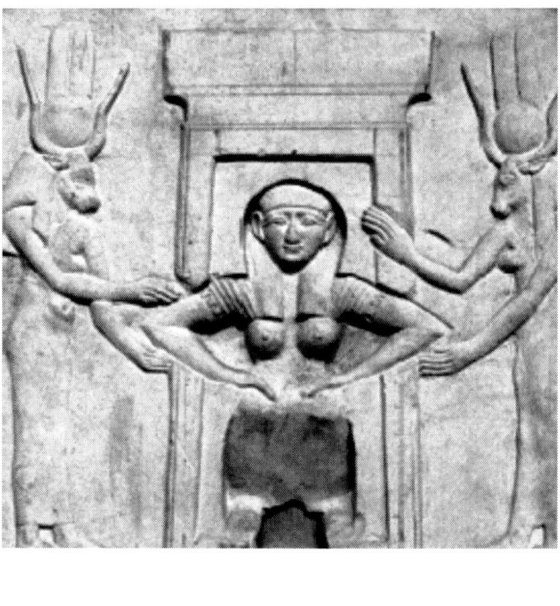

Figure 10
Egyptian Method of Midwife Delivery

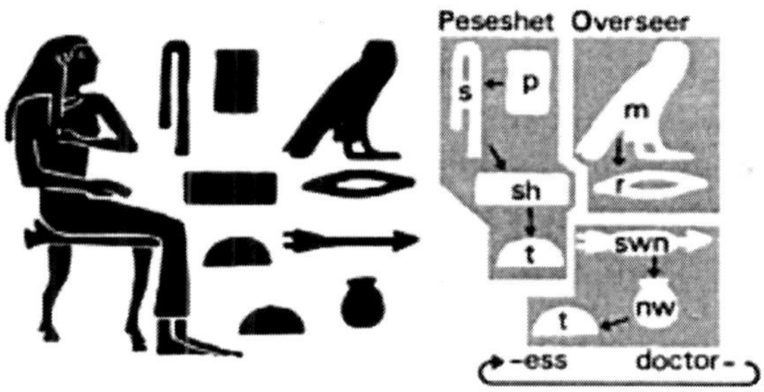

Figure 11
PESESHET (2,000 B.C.) The earliest known woman physician

Another physician whose name survives is that of Paneshi. This name indicates that he was a Nubian physician practicing in Egypt. It is an interesting question whether he was trained in Nubia or Egypt, though it is probable that since he was practicing in Egypt, he was trained there. This is further evidence of the symbiosis between Egypt and Nubia. The only other reference to a physician from beyond Egypt is of one Psammeticus, who, judging from his name came from Africa west of the Nile.

Our glimpse of the medical system of this ancient African civilization shows that it deserves its reputation as the best and most advanced of antiquity. Indeed, medicine as we know it today began in Egypt rather than Greece. So much of what is considered as the accomplishments of the modern world—science, technology, medicine, advanced cosmic knowledge—had already been discovered by the ancient inhabitants of the Nile Valley as long as 6,000 years ago.

A study of other African systems of medicine is more problematic however, because of the absence of surviving written records. Thus, most of what we know comes from the testimony of European missionaries whose contemptuous view of traditional culture was most pointed when writing about traditional medical practices. Nonetheless, it can be shown that the best of the traditional healers in various parts of Africa acquired a startling level of proficiency and, contrary to contemporary opinion, were not without a medical science.

It is pertinent to remember that Africa has been subjected to centuries of almost continuous political, social, and cultural disruption and that—among cultures that rely heavily on oral transmission of knowledge—a tremendous amount of knowledge has been lost. Thus, the state of traditional medicine today does not reflect the best of what the traditional doctors knew and surviving fragments of eyewitness reports—as shall be shown—indicate that they knew quite a lot.

Like ancient Egypt, all traditional African cultures had a magico-spiritual conception of disease. Thus in this setting, moral, social, or spiritual transgressions are likely to lead to illness because they create both individual and communal disharmony. Without the psycho-spiritual cure—without re-establishing this sensitive harmony—the medicinal cure is considered useless. The traditional practitioner is intimately acquainted with the psychic, social, and cultural nuances of his people and more than one commentator has acknowledged that the traditional doctor is often an expert psychotherapist, achieving results with his patients that conventional Western psychotherapy cannot.

Though there is no single paradigm of medical practice that applies to all of Africa, many of the essential features of the various traditional systems are comparable and even identical. Among the Mano of Liberia, for example, all children's diseases, all obstetrics, and all of the "everyday" complaints are handled by women, particularly the elderly women; surgery, bonesetting, and special diagnostic and therapeutic problems are handled almost exclusively by men. This is a pattern that repeats itself throughout Africa.

The approach to the patient can vary in different parts of Africa. In some societies, where the doctor is credited with paranormal insight, the physician may arrive at a diagnosis and prescribe treatment without questioning or examining the patient since he is supposed to know what is wrong by virtue of his special powers. However, other traditional doctors affect an approach toward physical diagnosis closer to our own:

> Many Western-trained donors concede that the traditional medical experts have a profound knowledge of the human body and anatomy. This is demonstrated by a usually careful diagnosis beginning with a history of the disease followed by a thorough physical examination... He palpates the different parts and looks for tender spots. He feels the beating of the heart, the position of the inner organs, checks the eyes and ears, and smells the mouth for bad breath.[29]

Most commentators have disparaged the traditional doctor's knowledge of anatomy and physiology. The Mano, however, have names for most of the major organs and know the difference between normal and abnormal anatomy.[30] Another author notes that the Banyoro of Uganda, renowned in the last century for their surgical skill, had a wide knowledge of anatomy.[31] A Hausa maneuver to test for impotence has been described:

> An individual is stripped and placed on a mat lying on his back. A pin or thorn is lightly rubbed over the inside of his thigh. If the scrotum or testicles do not move, the individual is considered impotent. There is a physiological basis for this procedure. The maneuver in effect tests the cremas-

29 Kiteme, K, "Doctor Still Makes House Calls", *Ebony,* p. 116.

30 Harley, G. W., *Native African Medicine,* London, Frank Cass, 1970, p. 41.

31 Davies, J. N., "Primitive Autopsies and Background to Scientific Medicine in Central Africa", *New York J Med,* 65:2831, 11/15/65.

> teric reflex. The cremaster muscle contracts and pulls the testicles upward on stimulation of the inside of the thigh.[32]

This passage belies the notion that African doctors were without a knowledge of some of the body's physiological processes. Moreover, Mano physicians—reputedly without an understanding of the body's cardiovascular system—knew that the conditions of anasarca and ascites were due to fluid overload and treated accordingly with diuretic preparations. These interesting fragments do not by themselves admit of a sophisticated anatomical or physiological knowledge but they hint at a greater degree of knowledge—perhaps in past ages—than has hitherto been recognized.

Some case studies of cultures in east-central Africa have brought to light some remarkable evidence revealing the presence of scientific medicine there. The practice of carrying out autopsies on patients dying of unknown causes among the Banyoro of Uganda and the Likundu of Central Africa has been described. Almost always these were carried out to detect a possible witchcraft etiology but may well have contributed to a more extensive knowledge of anatomy than previously supposed:

> The procedures for autopsying bodies under the Likundu culture have been reviewed, not for the purpose of considering the beliefs that impelled such procedures but to indicate that in some areas autopsies were frequently carried out and that they involved searching in the body, a search which might be casual and superificial but which in other cases might be prolonged and exacting and involved opening up and examining a variety of organs. These are precisely the circumstances under which considerable

32 Imperato, P. J., *African Folk Medicine.* Baltimore, York Press, 1979, p. 110.

knowledge of anatomy and pathology could be acquired by persons who, for any purpose, might wish to do so.[33]

Use of Natural Tetracycline in the Sudan 4th Century A.D.

Tetracycline-Labeled Human Bone from Ancient Sudanese Nubia (A.D. 350)

Abstract. *Nubian bone recovered from an X-group cemetery (A.D. 350 to 550) exhibits a pattern of fluorescence identical to that of modern tetracycline-labeled bone. When it is viewed under ultraviolet light at 490 angstroms, fluorophors are visible as a characteristic yellow-green fluorescence on surfaces that were actively mineralizing at the time of exposure. Contamination of stored grains provided the proper environment for cultivation of tetracycline-producing Streptomycetes. Evidence for exposure to antibiotics in an archeological population is relevant to studies of the evolution of R factors and to the interpretation of health and disease within the population.*[34]

An astonishing example comes to us from the northern Sudan among a people who lived there more than 1500 years ago. These people were intensive farmers, living along the banks of the Nile, whose bones were exhumed and sent to America as a consequence of the rise of the waters in Nubia after the completion of the Aswan High Dam. Purely by chance, a laboratory technician was examining the bones of 15 of these ancient Sudanese using a fluorescing technique that revealed very interesting patterns of "flashes" in the bones. Such intense fluorescent patterns in human bone are only caused by the presence of Tetracycline, a modern antibiotic second only to penicillin in its ubiquity. Tetracycline, after it is ingested and absorbed in the blood stream, is

33 Davies, op. cit., p. 2833.

34 Bassett, E.J., Keith, M.S., Armelagos, G.J., Martin, D.L., Villanueva, A.R., Science, 1980, Sept.26; 209(4464): 1532–4. *Tetracycline-labeled human bone from ancient Sudanese Nubia (A.D. 350)* DOI: 10.1126/science.7001623

taken up by actively mineralizing bone in a completely harmless way, making its presence in bone readily detectable.

How, then, does one explain the presence of a modern antibiotic in the bones of Sudanese farmers living more than 1500 years ago? Tetracycline, like all non-synthetic antibiotics, derives from a mold, in this case one belonging to the Streptomyces family. Streptomyces grows readily and abundantly in the soils of Upper Egypt and Nubia. What seems to have happened is that it grew easily on the stored grains of these agricultural Sudanese people living along the Nile. The real question is whether the subsequent ingestion of Streptomyces, i.e., natural Tetracycline, was accidental or purposeful. There are several strong clues: (1) all of the bones from the 15 individuals studied were free of periostitis, a bony inflammation caused by chronic infection; (2) the pattern

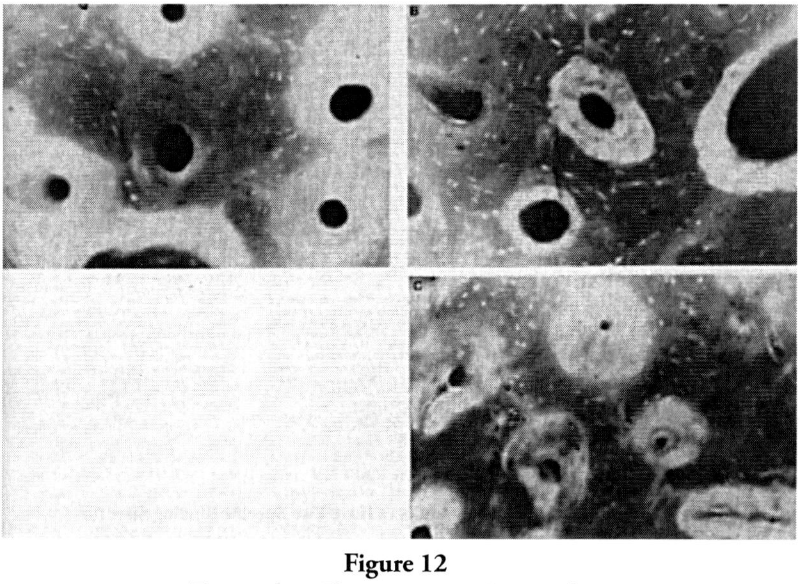

Figure 12
Tetracycline Fluorescence in Osteons from Sudanese Nubia (4th Century A.D.)

of fluorescence seen in these bones was of a kind only seen with therapeutic levels of Tetracycline; (3) grain is not usually eaten raw—it is milled, pounded, made into dough, and baked, which would have effectively destroyed any mold. Thus, we are driven to the conclusion that the anti-infective properties of this mold had been discovered by these Sudanese people, causing it to be collected from the grain and used purposely to treat infection. We know that many peoples around the world, including the ancient Egyptians, knew the therapeutic properties of penicillium mold; but this is the only known example anywhere of the use of Tetracycline in its natural form.[35]

Further, there is a report of a Banyoro king who commissioned a traditional doctor to travel around the countryside to investigate, describe, and search for a cure for sleeping sickness, which was ravaging the country at the time.[36] This event clearly indicates that a spirit of clinical investigation did exist among Banyoro physicians and probably among other traditional practitioners as well. In many parts of Africa, treatments were devised for new diseases like venereal disease and scrofula that were imported into Africa and this would presuppose some form of clinical investigation and experimentation.

Of further interest is the centuries-old practice of smallpox variolation which is carried out all over Africa. During an epidemic, material from the pustule of a sick person is scratched into the skin of unaffected persons with a thorn. In the majority of instances, there is no reaction and the persons inoculated are protected against smallpox. In some cases, the inoculation will

35 Ibid.

36 Davies, J. N., "The Development of 'Scientific' Medicine in the African Kingdom of Bunyoro-Kitara", *Med. Hist.*, 3:54, 1959.

produce a mild, non-fatal form of the disease which will also confer permanent immunity.

Historians like to say that the variolation technique was not truly vaccination in the modern sense. Also, that it was too dangerous to be of much efficacy because of the danger of inducing the disease. Anecdotal reports given to the author suggest that among many West African peoples where the technique was practiced, "attenuation" of the smallpox inoculum was attempted by heating or mixing with other substances. This procedure goes beyond "primitive" variolation. Centuries before Jenner, Africans had devised an effective immunization method against smallpox.

Cotton Mather, a Puritan clergyman and author living in the late 17th and early 18th centuries in New England learned the variolation method of inoculation from his slave, Onesimus, who may have come from the Gold Coast, or what is now Ghana. Mather wrote the following letter to the Royal Society of London in 1716:

> "Enquiring of my Negro-man Onesimus, who is a pretty Intelligent Fellow, Whether he ever had the Small-Pox; he answered, both, Yes, and No; and then told me, that he had undergone an Operation, which had given him something of the Small-Pox, and would forever preserve him from it, adding that it was often used among the Guramantese, & whoever had the Courage to use it, was forever free from

> the Fear of the Contagion. He described the Operation to me, and showed me in his Arm the Scar."[37, 38, 39]

Mather advocated the use of this inoculation during the smallpox outbreak of 1721, but at first, no one trusted information coming from an African slave. Mather was finally able to convince the physician, Zabdiel Boylston, to implement the procedure, and most of those who were inoculated lived. It became clear, as Mather spoke with enslaved Africans who had come from other parts of Africa, that the procedure had been widespread and well known throughout Africa and the Islamic world.[40]

It would seem that the traditional doctor had a firm grasp of some fundamental public health principles. In the urban areas of the Songhai Empire, soap was used, creating a high level of hygiene.[41]

In Liberia, the Mano developed an admirable quarantine system for smallpox. They were well aware of its contagiousness and set aside a "sick bush" for affected patients. This area was situated well away from the village and the patient was attended by only one person, who had already been infected with the disease; no one else was allowed to approach the area. The patient was put

37 Bell, Gregory, "Onesimus," in *African American Lives*, eds., Henry Louis Gates Jr. and Evelyn Brooks Higginbotham. Oxford: Oxford University Press, 2004, p. 641.
38 Koo, Kathryn, "Strangers in the House of God: Cotton Mather, Onesimus, and an Experiment in Christian Slaveholding," *Proceedings of the American Antiquarian Society*, 117 (2007): p.144
39 Wisecup, Kelly. "African Medical Knowledge, the Plain Style, and Satire in the 1721 Boston Inoculation Controversy." *Early American Literature* 46, no. 1 (2011): pp. 27–28.
40 Hayden, Christopher Ellis, "Of Medicine and Statecraft: Smallpox and Early Colonial Vaccination in French West Africa (Senegal-Guinea)." Evanston, IL: Northwestern University, PhD Dissertation, 2008, pp. 229–231.
41 Diop, C A, *PreColonial Black Africa, A comparative study of the political and social systems of Europe and Black Africa from antiquity to the formation of modern states,* translated by H Salemson, Brooklyn, NY, Lawrence Hill Books, p. 206.

on a careful diet and was rubbed with topical anaesthetic medications to prevent scratching which could lead to superinfection. When the illness ran its course, the area was burned. The "sick-bush" approach would do a modern epidemiologist proud.

In the area of surgery, the best evidence indicates that some African surgeons attained a level of skill comparable, and in some respects superior, to that of Western surgeons up to the 20th century. As in ancient Egypt, the bonesetter guilds were separate from those of the traditional doctors and were renowned for their skill. Some commentators, observing the bonesetters of today, feel that this reputation was somewhat inflated and the bonesetters' results were less than optimum by Western standards.[42] Yet other reports cite techniques that led to highly satisfactory results. Mano bonesetters treated a patient with a thigh fracture by placing him in the loft of a house allowing the affected leg to dangle free with a heavy stone attached. This was a very effective traction method and once the fracture was reduced, it was immobilized with a tight splint.[43] In addition, the patient was encouraged to exercise a fractured leg and we know today that new bone is laid down more rapidly over the fracture site when there is some exercise of the limb. Bonesetters in other parts of Africa would dig a deep pit for the purpose of exercising traction on a fractured limb and in East Africa, the bonesetters reduced fractures and dislocations by manual manipulation and traction. These examples indicate that the bonesetters' reputation was not entirely undeserved.

In many areas, especially where wars or battles occurred frequently, the traditional physician was particularly adept in

42 Ibid., pp. 55–6.
43 Harley, op. cit., p. 95.

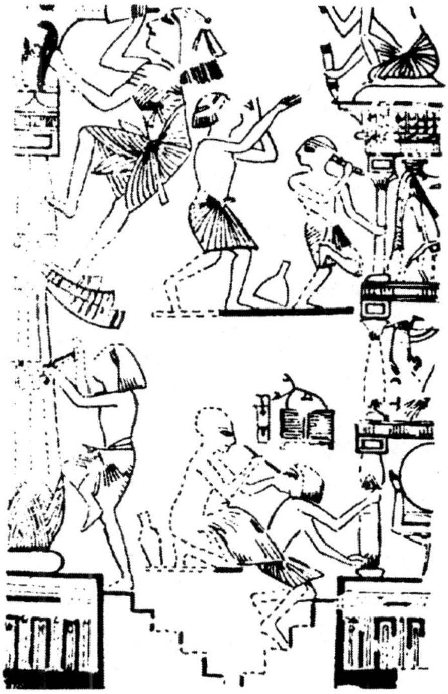

Figure 13

A person treats another workman's eye by means of a sticklike instrument (lower frame), either removing a foreign body or instilling drops.

treating traumatic wounds. One report describes the treatment of an open wound by the following method: plant juices with antiseptic properties were squeezed into the open wound, a red hot metal tip was used to cauterize bleeding points and burn away damaged tissue, the wound edges were closed with a tough thorn, an awl, and fibrous suture, and a fiber mat was wrapped tightly around the wound to prevent bleeding. The wound was never closed until the bleeding had been stopped.[44] In another

44 Ibid., p. 221.

documented instance, a native surgeon successfully resected part of a patient's lung to remove a penetrating arrowhead.[45] In the Congo, a native surgeon was seen using stiff elephant hairs to probe for and successfully remove a bullet.[46] In Nigeria, a man who had had his abdomen ripped open by an elephant was treated by the doctor by replacing the intestines in the abdominal cavity, securing them in place with a calabash covering, and finally suturing together the overlying abdominal and skin. Not only did the man recover but was soon back working on a road gang.[47] In the testimony of one author:

> Witch doctors of many tribes perform operations for cataract. They squeeze the juice from the leaves of an alkaloid-containing plant directly into the eye to desensitize it, then push the cataract aside with a sharp stick. A surprising number of these cases turn out successfully.[48]

In East Africa, Masai surgeons were known to successfully treat pleurisy and pneumonia by creating a partial collapse of the lung by drilling holes into the chest of the sufferer.[49]

We have already noted that trepanation or craniotomy had been practiced in northern Africa at least since the end of the neolithic period. The technique may have undergone even greater development in East Africa, particularly among the Kisii of western Kenya. Indications for the operation include chronic headache, increased intracranial pressure, and skull fracture. The technique can (but does not always) involve boring down

45 Ibid., p. 222.
46 Ibid.
47 Ibid.
48 Thompson, E. E., "Primitive Medical Lore and Witchcraft", *Bull Med. Libr. Ass.*, 53:89–90, 1/65.
49 Johnston, H, *The Uganda Protectorate.* London, Hutchinson & Co., 2:750, 1902.

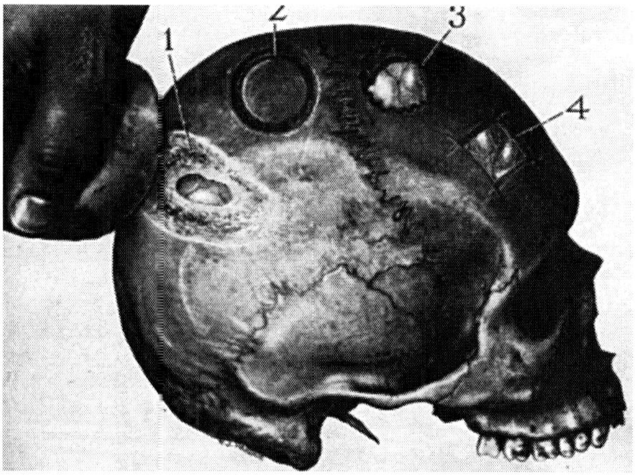

Figure 14
Techniques of Craniotomy Kisii Province of Kenya

through the skull to the pia mater. Traditional trepanation is still practiced among the Kisii, and a survey of the practice done in 1957–58 showed that somewhere between 500–1000 operations of this kind had been performed in the region with about a 1% mortality rate. One operator had apparently performed over 100 such procedures without one single fatality![50] [51]

Cheikh Anta Diop describes the treatment of soldiers in Senegal wounded by gunfire:

> War wounds were treated by extracting the bullets or shrapnel, then cauterizing the wound with a mixture of boiling oil and clean sand, before sewing it up. It thus happened that some soldiers still had, after recovery, lumps of matter

50 Margetts, Edward L, "Trepanation of the Skull by the Medicine-Men of Primitive Cultures, with Particular Reference to Present-Day Native East African Practice," Diseases in Antiquity, edited by Brothwell D and Sandison, A T. Springfield: , Charles C. Thomas, 1967, p.690.
51 See also Grounds J G, "Trephining of the Skull Amongst the Kisii," East African Journal of Medicine.(35), 1957, pp. 369–73 for discussion of 500+ cases of trepanation in Kenya with only 6 deaths.

> (sand) which had remained under the skin. It seems no one ever thought of removing them. That process is called *rukâb* in Wolof.[52]

Other examples of surgery also show exceptional skill. The Masai of Kenya and Tanzania also have the capability of successfully performing limb amputations, even devising prostheses for severed limbs. They treat chronic pneumonia with pulmonary resections, and drain liver abscesses.[53]

It is pertinent to now consider one of the most remarkable examples of African surgery ever documented. This is an eyewitness account by a missionary doctor named Felkin of a Caesarean section performed by a Banyoro surgeon in Uganda in 1879:

> The patient was a healthy-looking primipara (first pregnancy) of about twenty years of age and she lay on an inclined bed, the head of which rested against the side of the hut. She was half-intoxicated with banana wine, was quite naked and was tied down to the bed by bands of bark cloth over the thorax and thighs. Her ankles were held by a man... while another man stood on her right steadying her abdomen... the surgeon was standing on her left side holding the knife aloft and muttering an incantation. He then washed his hands and the patient's abdomen first with banana wine and then water. The surgeon made a quick cut upwards from just above the pubis to just below the umbilicus severing the whole abdominal wall and uterus so that amniotic fluid escaped. Some bleeding points in the abdominal wall were touched with red hot irons. The surgeon completed the uterine incision, the assistant helping by holding up the sides of the abdominal wall with his hand and hooking two

52 op. cit., Diop, p. 206.

53 Ackernecht, Erwin H, "Primitive Surgery," in Diseases in Antiquity, op. cit., p.640

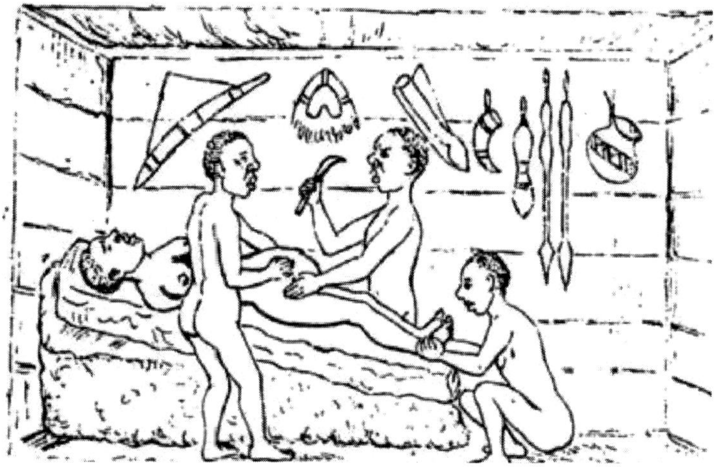

Figure 15
Illustration from Dr. R. W. Felkin's description of the Caesarean section. Edinburgh Medical Journal, 1884.

> fingers into the uterus. The child was removed, the cord cut, and the child was handed to an assistant."[54]

The report goes on to say that the surgeon squeezed the uterus until it contracted, dilated the cervix from inside with his fingers (to allow post-partum blood to escape), removed clots and the placenta from the uterus, and then *sparingly* used red hot irons to seal the bleeding points. A porous mat was tightly secured over the wound and the patient turned over to the edge of the bed to permit drainage of any remaining fluid. The peritoneum, the abdominal wall, and the skin were approximated back together and secured with seven sharp spikes. A root paste was applied over the wound and a bandage of cloth was tightly wrapped around it. Within six days, all the spikes were removed. Felkin

54 Davies, The Development..., op. cit., pp. 50–1.

observed the patient for 11 days and when he left, mother and child were alive and well.[55]

In Scotland, Lister had pioneered antiseptic surgery just two years prior to this event but universal application of his methods in the operating rooms of Europe was still years away. Caesarean sections were performed *only* under the most desperate circumstances and *only* to save the life of the infant. A Caesarean section to save the lives of both mother and child was unheard of in Europe nor are there records of such a procedure among the great civilizations of antiquity. As one commentator has said:

> The whole conduct of the operation as Felkin described it suggests a skilled long-practiced surgical team at work conducting a well-tried and familiar operation with smooth efficiency and unhurried skill... Lister's team in London could hardly have performed with greater smoothness.[56]

Not only did the surgeon understand the sophisticated concepts of anaesthesia and antisepsis but also demonstrated advanced surgical technique. In his sparing use of the cautery iron, for example, he showed that he knew tissue damage could result from its overuse. The operation was without question a landmark, reflecting the best in African surgery.

African midwives possessed a good understanding of some fundamental obstetric and pediatric principles. Mano midwives pulled repeatedly at the breasts of women in labour, a maneuver which induces the release of oxytocin from the pituitary gland – a stimulator of uterine contractions. They sometimes took laboring mothers upon their backs, walking around with

55 Ibid.
56 Ibid., p. 52.

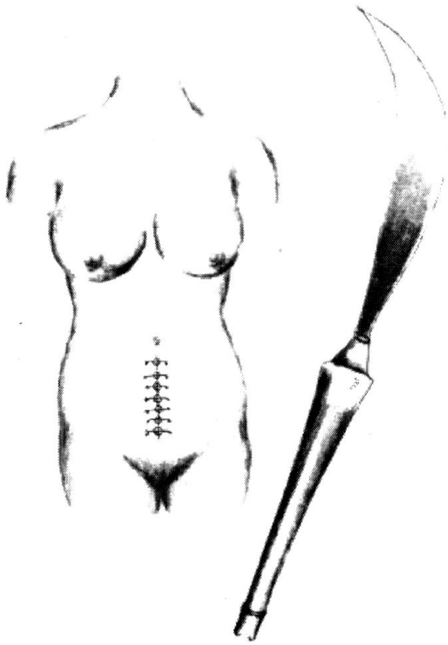

Figure 16

Knife used in the Caesarean section described by Felkin in 1879; also, illustration of post-Caesarean wound closure from Felkin's description. Edinburgh Medical Journal, 1884. Redrawn for publication by Sylvia Bakos.

them and shaking them. This undoubtedly had the effect of causing the cervix to dilate and the head to engage, thus facilitating labor.[57] Some Bantu midwives were known to use Indian hemp during labor for its sedative properties. Newborn babies and infants were taken and exposed to the sun for a period of each day "to make them strong." A condition known as physiologic jaundice is common in newborns. With their immature liver, newborns may not be able to eliminate bilirubin, giving the skin a yellowed appearance. One of the treatments for this

57 See "Ambulation Versus Oxytocin for Improved Labor", *Family Practice Recertification,* 3(11): 11, 11/81.

SCENES OF TRADITIONAL MIDWIFERY
Eastern Nigeria (Ibo)

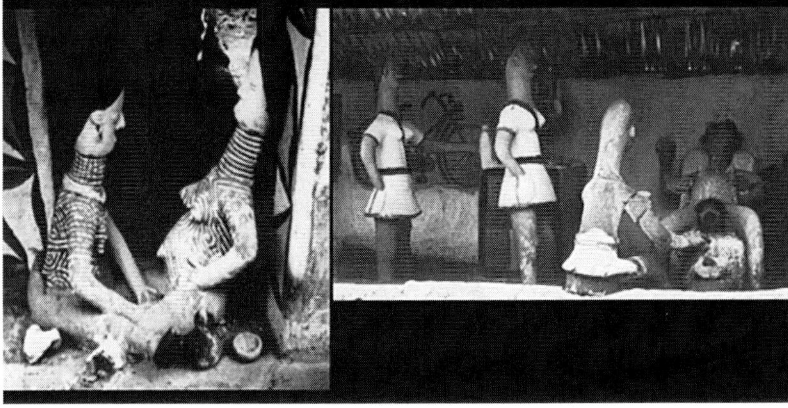

condition is phototherapy. The light breaks down the bilirubin molecules, allowing them to be excreted in urine or stool. Exposure to the sun for short periods would have helped this condition in traditional Africa. Sun exposure would have also helped to prevent rickets, which, according to one author is rare among Mano children.[58] In addition, these women healers recognized the causes of malnutrition and retarded development, putting such children on special diets high in vitamins and carbohydrates with favorable results.[59] In Uganda, in an area where there is a high incidence of dystocia (retarded labour), the midwives have preparations which stimulate uterine contractions.[60]

58 Harley, op. cit., p. 64.

59 Ibid.

60 Kamatenesi-Mugisha M, Oryem-Origa H, Medicinal plants used to induce labour during childbirth in western Uganda, *Journal of Ethnopharmacology*, Elsevier, 3 January 2007.

Traditional African cultures have an abundant materia medica. The Zulus, for example, are reputed to know the medicinal uses of some 700 plants.[61] Ouabain, capsicum, physostigmine, kola, and calabar beans are just a few of the substances from the African materia medica that have made their way into the Western pharmacopeia.[62] Certain Bantu-speaking peoples use the bark of *Salix capensis* (willow) to treat the musculoskeletal complaints of rheumatism.[63] This family of plants yields salicylic acid, the active ingredient in aspirin, a sovereign remedy the world over for musculoskeletal pains. Kaolin, the active ingredient in Kaopectate is used in Mali to combat diarrhea. Caffeine-containing kola nuts are chewed all over Africa for their stimulating and fatigue-combating properties. To combat snakebite, plants containing ouabain and strichnine are used. The former is a heart stimulant and therefore useful against cardiotoxic venoms and the latter is a nerve tonic, useful against neurotoxic venoms. In Nigeria, in 1979, the rootbark *Annona senegalensis* was found to possess strong anticancer properties.[64] Even earlier, in 1969, herbal preparations that were used in Nigeria to treat skin infections were found to have definite bacteriocidal activity against gram-positive bacteria, the very organisms that cause skin infections.[65] There was an interesting case in 1925 of an eminent Nigerian in England who was suffering from severe psychotic

61 Bryant, A. T., *Zulu Medicine and Medicine-Men. Capetown, C.* Struik, 1966, p. 84.

62 Thompson, op. cit., p. 83.

63 Hewat, M, *Bantu Folklore.* Cape Town, T. Maskew Miller, 1906, p. 62.

64 Durodola, J. I., "Contribution of Traditional Medicine to the Chemotherapy of Cancer", Niger Med. J., 9(5):616, 5–6/79.

65 Malcolm, S. A., Sofowara E. A., "Antimicrobial Activity of Selected Nigerian Folk Remedies and Their Constituent Plants", *Lloydia,* 32:512–7, 12/69.

episodes not amenable to treatment by English doctors. A traditional doctor from Nigeria was summoned who was able to relieve the patient of his symptoms with decoctions made from a rauwolfia root.[66] The *Rauwolfia* family of plants is the source of modern-day Reserpine, first used as a major tranquilizer to treat severe psychosis but then became one of the first anti-hypertensive medications.[67]

Traditional doctors in Africa have effective remedies against intestinal parasites, vomiting, skin ulcers, rashes, catarrh, convulsions, tumours, venereal disease, bronchitis, conjunctivitis, urethral stricture and many other complaints. The list of effective drugs in the African pharmacopeia is too extensive to elucidate here but suffice to say that traditional doctors in Africa had and have effective remedies against intestinal parasites, vomiting, skin ulcers, rashes, catarrh, convulsions, tumours, venereal disease, bronchitis, conjunctivitis, urethral stricture and many other complaints.

The Neem tree, *Azadirachta indica* grows throughout Africa, and traditional therapists have used its leaves and bark to treat malaria and musculo-skeletal pain. Decoctions of this plant have been shown to reduce the parasite count in malaria-infected mice.[68] Moreover, tinctures derived from *Azadirachta indica* have shown greater anti-inflammatory activity than aspirin. In Ghana, the herb, *Combretum mucronatum,* commonly used there to treat guinea worm infestation, was found to cause complete extrusion of the worms in 43 or 44 patients in a non-blinded study.[69] If

66 Aikman, L, "Nature's Gift to Medicine", *National Geographic,* 146(3):428, 9/74.
67 Sofowara, Abayomi, *Medicinal Plants and Traditional Medicine in Africa*, New York: John Wiley and Sons Limited, 1982, pp. 75–6.
68 Sofowara, Abayomi, *Medicinal Plants and Traditional Medicine in Africa,* New York: John Wiley and Sons Limited, 1982, p.76
69 Ibid., p. 76

this herb (and others) could be grown, harvested, and distributed over a broad area, one could imagine the tremendous savings in foreign exchange that would ensue once freed from the necessity of importing anti-parasitic medications from abroad.

There are several well-known anti-diabetic treatments used by traditional therapists throughout Africa. One of the most effective is derived from the plant species *bridelia ferruginea.* In three instances reported in one study, elevated blood sugars returned to normal after 12 weeks on a regimen of 3-times-daily oral intake of a decoction of this plant.[70] The chewing stick, *zanthoxylum zanthoxylides,* is used throughout West Africa to clean teeth. Not only does the chewing of the stick release non-toxic, anti-microbial juices that inhibit tooth decay, but *zanthoxylum* also prevents sickling in a sickle cell-endemic region of Africa.[71] In Nigeria, the plant, *Moringa pterygospermia* has been used to treat scurvy, as this species of Moringa is also rich in vitamin C.[72]

Many native plants, have more than one application. The famed baobab tree has been used to treat malaria, tuberculosis, fever, microbial infections, diarrhea, anemia, toothache, and dysentery. In addition, oil from the seeds has been found to beautify the skin, smoke from burned leaves makes an insect repellent, and the water solutions of the bark soothe inflammation and swelling. This tree is so important to life in a dry, hot climate, that it has spiritual significance to the people, as well.[73]

70 Ibid., p.77

71 Ibid., p. 218

72 Liaso, K., Geldenhuys, C.J., Chirwa, P.W. *Traditional uses and local perspectives on baobab (Adansonia digitata) population structure by selected ethnic groups in Northern Namibia, South African Journal of Botany,* Vol. 113, Nov. 2017, pp.449–456.

73 op. cit., Sofowara, p. 71

Ocimum gratissimum, is a common anti-diarrhetic medication whose efficacy has been confirmed by laboratory experiments. The tests show that decoctions of *ocimum* relax the ileum and jejunum of guinea pigs.[74] Moreover, it is extremely effective as an insect repellent. For that reason, it is planted near houses in Africa. Another plant with multiple applications is *pergularia daemia* which is used traditionally as a post-partum uterine contracting agent, a post-circumcision anesthetic, and as a topical treatment for external wounds and abscesses. Laboratory studies have shown that all of these uses of the plant are empirically justified on the basis of their demonstrated effects, as well as the pharmacoactive constituents of the plant. [75]

Finally, in East and West Africa, the herb, *Euphorbia hirta L.* is used widely to treat asthma and bronchitis. In fact, its anti-asthmatic, anti-bronchitic properties are so well established, that it is often called simply the "asthma herb." In the laboratory, *euphorbia* has shown marked broncho-dilating and expectorant actions entirely consistent with its use in asthma and bronchitis.[76]

Recently a study has shown that a traditional medicinal herb growing in Senegal, Momordica balsamina, has been shown to be effective in reducing viral loads in patients with HIV-1. The use of Momordica balsamina, which is given in the form of a tea to patients, could be a cost effective treatment given the high cost of HIV medications in other parts of the world.[77]

74 Ibid., pp. 199–202

75 Ibid., pp. 209–13

76 Ackernecht, Erwin H., "Primitive Surgery" in *Diseases in Antiquity,* op. cit., p. 640.

77 Mahfuz Khan, et al. Anti-human immunodefciency virus-1 activity of MoMo30 protein isolated from the traditional African medicinal plant Momordica balsamina, *Virology Journal* (2023) 20:50 https://doi.org/10.1186/s12985-023-02010-5

These are at least two documented instances of Europeans benefiting from the ministrations of the traditional physician. In the last century, a Khoisan doctor cured a European woman dying of sepsis that the European doctor could not treat. In Swaziland, a European doctor, dying of dysentery, was cured by a native physician.[78] Moreover, the native physicians in this area were so skilled at treating Typhoid Fever that the European doctors used their decoctions for the same purpose.[79]

Increasing study of the traditional materia-medica of sub-Saharan Africa reveals that traditional therapists, from antiquity to the present, discovered and utilized the pharmacotherapeutic properties of hundreds of native plants. We might add parenthetically that the conventional separation of "herbalism" from modern pharmacology is somewhat artificial; modern pharmacopeia includes numerous products derived wholly or in part from traditional medicinal herbs from around the world.

This chapter has attempted to show that the traditional doctors of Africa from the earliest times had a high level of medical and surgical skill, certainly much more than they have been given credit for. It is to be hoped that more substantive and careful investigations will be carried out among the traditional healers of Africa before Western-style medicine supplants them entirely.

78 Harley, op. cit., p. 250.
79 Hewat, op. cit., p. 79.

CHAPTER TWO

Imhotep the Physician: Archetype of the Great Man

Imhotep, "Father of Medicine"

No individual more fully embodies the highest and finest of Egyptian medicine than the figure of Imhotep. Sir William Osler, prominent Canadian physician of the late 19th and early 20th centuries, called him "the first figure of a physician to stand out clearly from the mists of antiquity."[1] In truth, he is the world's first universal genius of whom we have any knowledge. As vizier to the pharaoh Djoser, he was a statesman of the first rank; as designer and builder of the world's first great edifice in stone, the step-pyramid of Saqqara, he was an architect of transcendant genius; as the renowned purveyor of wise sayings and parables, he was the epitome of the sage; and finally, as the divinely-gifted physician he was accorded that rarest of honours in ancient Egypt, deification as the god of healing. In spite of this, there are those who question whether Imhotep

1 Osler, William, *The Evolution of Modern Medicine*, A series of lectures delivered at Yale University on the Silliman Foundation in April, 1913. The Project Gutenberg Etext of The Evolution of Modern Medicine, Etext #1566, Dec. 1998.

actually was a physician. Jonckeere, when compiling his list of 103 Egyptian physicians mentioned by name in the inscriptions, omitted Imhotep because of the dearth of contemporary witnesses to the fact.[2] Yet within a century after his death, he was venerated by Men-kau-ra (Mycerinus), third pharaoh of the 4th dynasty, as a healer[3] and his powers as a physician made such an impression on succeeding generations both in and out of Egypt, that he was eventually deified in his own country and identified with the healing god Asclepios by the Greeks from the 6th century B.C. on. If we use Jonckeere's yardstick, we would have to eliminate Hippocrates from the ranks of physicians because next to nothing is known about his actual life or healing accomplishments. The books attributed to him are almost all written by later followers and even the famous Hippocratic Oath was not written by him but by professional disciples at a time long after his death.[4] Yet no one doubts that Hippocrates existed, that he practiced the healing art, or that he was a clinician of unusual gifts. Hippocrates is, if anything, a more shadowy figure than Imhotep, but his life and healing work are not open to question. Neither is that of Imhotep. Hippocrates, who is customarily accorded the title "Father of Medicine," i.e., the practitioner in antiquity most responsible for introducing "clinical" or "scientific" medicine to the world, was himself said to be descended from a long line of "Asclepiads," that is, devotees of the Greek healing god

2 See Majno, G., *The Healing Hand: Man and Woundin the Ancient World,* Cambridge: Harvard University Press, 1982, p. 480, n. 52.

3 Hurry, J. B., *Imhotep,* New York: AMS Press, Inc., 1978, pp. 45–6.

4 Bogdonoff, M.D., et al, editors, "Introduction", *The Aphorisms of Hippocrates,* Birmingham: Classics of Medicine Library, 1982, pp. 3–7.

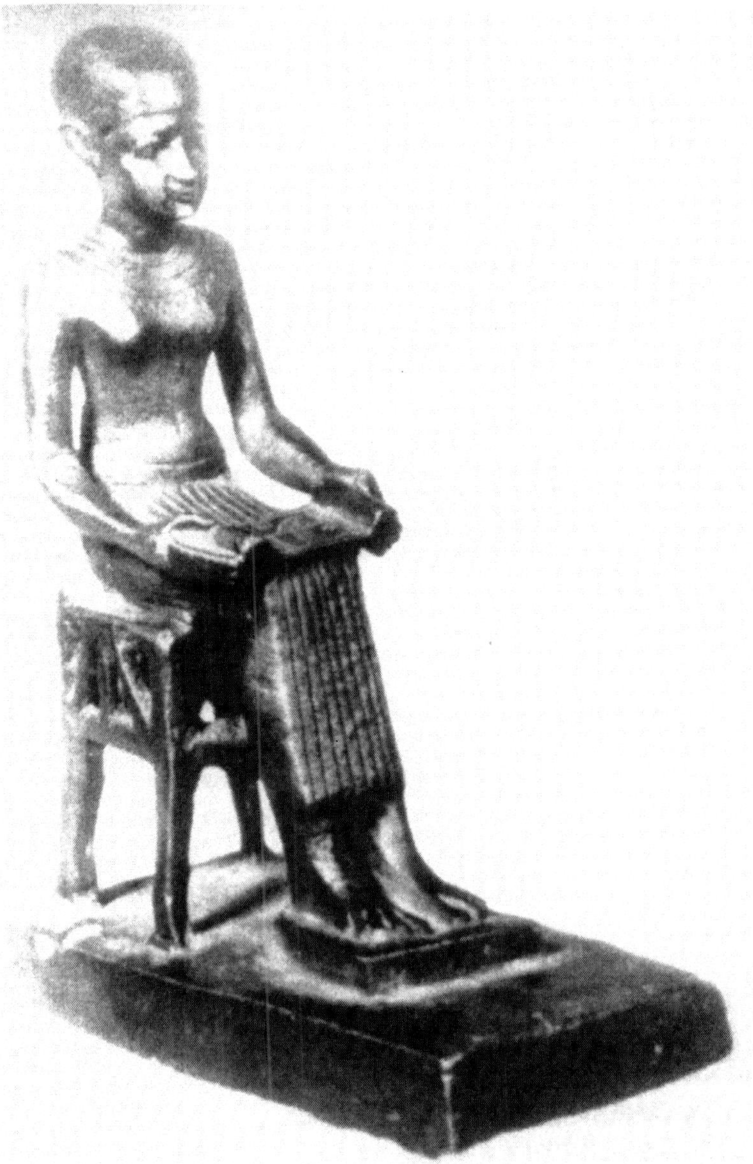

Figure 1
Imhotep: Physician, Sage, and Scribe.

Asclepios. In the famous oath ascribed to him—but which he did not compose—he is made to swear by the important healing gods of Greece, including Asclepios.[5] It is clear that neither Hippocrates nor later members of his school forswore "priestly medicine," since they were in the habit of referring patients to the healing temples of Asclepios for special cures.[6] Moreover, by swearing by Asclepios in the Oath, the members of the Hippocratic school were in fact swearing by Imhotep, since the two were synonymous in the Greek mind. The reputed clinical or scientific primacy of the Hippocratic school was finally laid to rest in 1930 when J. H. Breasted translated the Edwin Smith Papyrus, a document whose original antedates Hippocrates by over 2500 years. The diagnostic, prognostic, and therapeutic methodology revealed in this document demonstrated that even in our own day, our physicians have not surpassed the clinical acumen of the priest-physicians of the Nile Valley, of whom Imhotep was the epitome. The Egyptian priests told Solon, the great Greek lawgiver, that the Greeks were "as children" compared to the Egyptians;[7] and it is clear from what has just been said that Hippocrates in no way merits the title "Father of Medicine", either by virtue of his antiquity or the level of his scientific thought. If such a title belongs to anyone, it belongs to Imhotep. In spite of their propaganda in favour of Hippocrates, the Greeks themselves knew this. Galen is merely the most eminent and most famous of Greek physicians who

5 The Hippocratic Oath opens as follows: "I swear by Apollo, the physician, by Aesculapius, by Hygeia, and by Panacea".

6 Majno, op. cit., p. 201. In one of the Hippocratic books, the physician says, "The gods are the real physicians..."

7 Plato, *Timaeus,* translated by Desmond Lee, New York: Penguin Books, 1979, p. 35.

continued to travel to the temple of Imhotep in the early centuries A.D. in search of medical knowledge.[8]

Imhotep, The Man

As will be seen later on, there was a substantial corpus of myth, legend, and symbol that grew up around the figure of Imhotep, as with other extraordinary men in history, and there are only a few fragments of true biographical detail that can be extracted from the welter of legendary tradition that surrounds his name. His father was Kanofer who preceded Imhotep as a distinguished architect in the service of pharaoh, and his mother was Khreduonkh who was from a high-born family that originated in Mendes. He was born on the 31st of May in a suburb of Memphis called Ankhtaui ("Life of the Two Lands") and served as prime minister, chief scribe, ritualist, and architect under the pharaoh Djoser of the IIIrd dynasty. Mastery of any one of these would have marked him as a great man but he seems to have excelled in all. But even these extraordinary talents appeared to have been overshadowed by his gifts as a physician. Hurry, who has written the best English-language monograph on Imhotep, described the stages by which Imhotep was elevated to the status of healing deity; for within a hundred years after his death he was venerated—though not worshipped—as the Great Physician.[9] He held this status for more than 2000 years until just before the Persian conquest when he was elevated to the status of full-fledged deity, possibly under Greek or other

8 Hurry, op. cit., p. 115. Hurry also states that "many Egyptian drugs and prescriptions were copied by the Greeks and in due course were incorporated into the Pharmacopeias of other nations".
9 See note 3.

non-Egyptian influence. Herodotus asserts that at no time during the proper history of Egypt was a mortal man ever deified. Even the divinity of the pharaoh was a mythical construct designed to cement the ties between earth and heaven, human and divine. However, if Herodotus is to be relied on, no non-pharaoh was ever paid divine honors, whereas the Greeks were very much in the habit of deifying mortal men of heroic stature. The profound veneration that surrounded the name and figure of Imhotep in Egypt in the 6th century when the Greeks made their first significant penetration into Egypt must have made a marked impression on them—as did all things Egyptian—for they forthwith declared their own healing god Asclepios to be a form of Imhotep. It is during Ptolemaic times (332–30 B.C.) that Imhotep, now fully deified, advances to the front rank of the gods in Egypto-Hellenic pantheon.

The existence of Imhotep and his relation to the pharaoh Djoser is attested to by a statue of Djoser, found near the step-pyramid of Saqqara in 1926, on which Imhotep's name is inscribed. In addition, the Egyptian architect Khnum-ib-re ("opening to the heart of Khnum"), living around 495 B.C., left an inscription which records the names of 25 of his remote ancestors, all of whom were fathers and sons and all of whom were master-builders.[10] The pedigree, according to Hurry, covers a span of 800 years, beginning with Kanofer, the father of Imhotep, with Imhotep second. Imhotep, in this record, is described as "the chief of works, both of the South and of the North-land, governor of the capital and vizier, chief ritual priest of Zozer, the King of Upper and Lower Egypt, the son of Kanofer, chief of works of the South-land of

10 Hurry, op. cit., pp. 193–5.

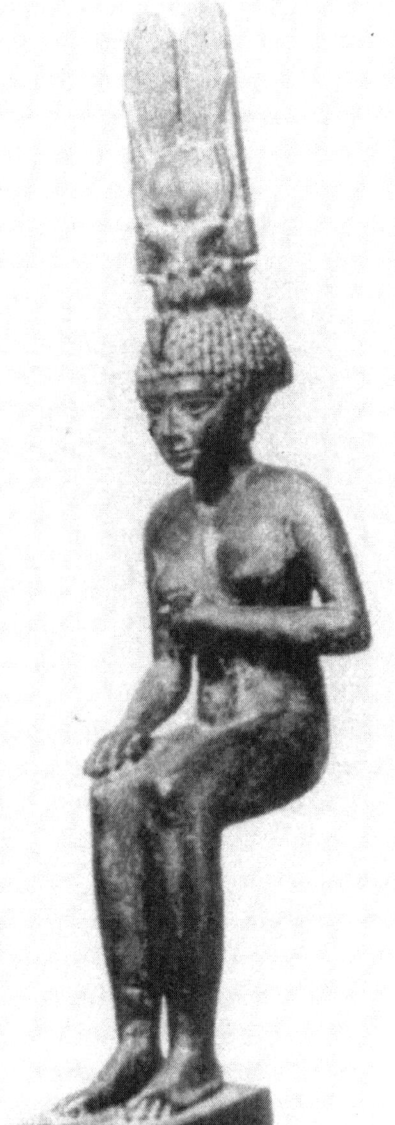

Figure 2
Khreduonkh, mother of Imhotep.

the North-land".[11] Gerald Massey called Imhotep "the Egyptian Solomon",[12] and with good reason, for Imhotep was without peer as an architect and builder. Architecture was a sacred science in Egypt embodying the highest in Egyptian scientific and religious thought. Thus, the parallel between Imhotep, builder of the temple, and Solomon, builder of the temple, is quite pertinent. Solomon is "Selmeh" in Hebrew. Looking at this word—"Selmeh"—through the Egyptian language, it can be analyzed in the following manner: "sel"="ser" ("l" and "r" are linguistically interchangeable), and "meh" gives "meh" in Egyptian unchanged. The Egyptian word "ser(l)" means "chief, noble, princely, royal"; the Egyptian word "meh" means "cubit," which brought together as "Selmeh" gives, in Egyptian, "the royal cubit."[13] Now the royal cubit was *the* unit of measure used in the construction of all important buildings and temples and therefore was the sign—par excellence—of the builder. Moreover, Imhotep's divine father Ptah was the "god of the cubit" because he too was the Divine Mason. From this point of view, then, Massey's linking Imhotep and Solomon is entirely accurate. Modern Freemasons, therefore, do not seem to go back far enough when they designate Solomon as the (legendary) founder of their order.

Imhotep's relationship with the pharaoh Djoser is made more revealing by a tradition which curiously echoes the Biblical story of Joseph. This is the so-called Legend of the Seven Years Famine which was found inscribed on a granite rock on the island of Sehel

11 Ibid.

12 Massey, G., *Ancient Egypt: Light of the World,* New York: Samuel Weiser, 1970, p. 365.

13 Budge, E. A. W., *Egyptian Hieroglyphic Dictionary,* 2 volumes, New York: Dover Publications, 1978.

just south of Aswan during the Ptolemaic period. Hurry thinks that the legend itself dates from as early as the IIIrd dynasty. The Legend describes a period during Djoser's reign in which the Nile seven times failed to reach its normal flood height, precipitating and prolonging a terrible famine in Egypt. The Nile flood was thought to be controlled by the ram-god Khnum, a Nubian deity whose shrine was situated at Elephantine in Egyptian Nubia. In this time of peril, Djoser turned to Imhotep who thereupon consulted the sacred books locked away in the deepest, most inaccessible regions of the temple. From this Imhotep was able to reveal to the king how he might approach and propitiate Khnum. After paying a personal visit to the temple of Khnum and performing prayers and sacrifices, the god appeared to the king in a dream and promised to release the flood once again so that Egypt might be spared any further famine. With the return of the Nile flood, the overjoyed king endowed the temple of Khnum with seventy miles of the richest land bordering the Nile and heaped munificent gifts and benefices upon the temple. It is hard indeed to determine how much of this reflects an actual occurrence. There was a tendency in Ptolemaic times to extol and romanticize old Egypt, which is one reason for Imhotep's rise to prominence during the period. However, the Ptolemies had access to all the archives of ancient Egypt and it is from these that many of the traditions that crop up around Imhotep are derived. Whether, as is often the case in such matters, they were embellished in such a way as to add lustre to Imhotep's name to justify his deification is impossible to say. It is, however, difficult not to presume that there was at least a hard kernel of truth in such traditions which give us fleeting glimpses of Imhotep the man.

Sage of Sages

One thing that comes through clearly in pre-Hellenic traditions concerning Imhotep is that he was a sage and adept of the first magnitude. His name is linked very closely with other legendary Egyptian sages such as Hardedef who lived in the IVth dynasty, Kegemni who lived at the end of the IIIrd dynasty, Ptah-hotep who lived during the Vth dynasty, and finally and most of all, Amenhotep son of Hapu who lived during the 18th dynasty. This latter, like Imhotep, was deified during Ptolemaic times and was considered, in effect, a reincarnation of Imhotep.[14] Imhotep as the purveyor of ageless oral wisdom comes through in the Song of the Harper where he is linked with sage Hardedef:

> I have heard the discourses of Imhotep and Hardedef, with whose words men speak everywhere...[15]

In these simple phrases Imhotep as philosopher and teacher shows himself unmistakably. In addition, particularly since we know him as a priest and ritualist, Imhotep's reputation would to a great extent rest on his command over the forces of nature, i.e., as a "magician". Whatever the modern prejudice about such things, the ability to control the forces of nature was a universally accepted idea in antiquity and all the great sages and adepts were acknowledged to have possessed such abilities. Indeed, it is difficult to understand the extraordinary reverence paid to men such as Imhotep and Amenhotep son of Hapu in the absence of such abilities. The wonder-works of Moses and the miracles of Jesus are in this vein and it is such powers that cast an aura of divinity around such persons. It is not too much to say that Imhotep is the

14 Hurry, op. cit., pp. 73, 103.
15 Ibid., pp. 24–5.

recognizably first in a line that leads directly to the later "prophets", "avatars", and "great souls" which would include Moses, Zoroaster, Gautama, and Jesus. In the Egypto-Hellenic world he was plainly seen as such.

Imhotep's name in Egyptian was "Iu-em-hetep" which means "he who comes in peace". This name became Hellenized as "Imouthes" and conventionalized in modern times as "Imhotep". Gerald Massey was of the opinion that Imhotep was a pre-existing deity and that the historical man of the IIIrd dynasty was merely his namesake. This is rather obscure when it is considered that in the Old Kingdom, the trinity of Memphis consisted of Ptah, Sekhmet, and Nefer-Tum; only in the late period does Iu-em-hetep or Imhotep supplant Nefer-Tum as the third member of the Memphis triad. There is, perhaps, another way of looking at the matter. Osiris, Buddha, and Christ—each was a deified man, but it is clear that each was the namesake of a divine being that preexisted the historical individual. The author has remarked elsewhere that a vast corpus of pre-extant saviour and resurrection mythology coalesced around the man Joshua ben Pandera ("Joshua son of the Panther") early in the Piscean Age to create the figure of Jesus the Christ, Son of God.[16] According to Massey, the Christhood had already existed in Egypt for 10,000 years as the "krst"—"kristos" in Greek—the anointed mummy who in different phases was Seker and then Osiris, the sign and symbol of resurrection.[17] Something similar seems to have occurred with respect to Osiris and Buddha. Abbe Amelineau discovered the tomb of Osiris in 1897, who subsequently was shown to be

16 See Finch, C., "Studies in Kamite Origins: The Works of Gerald Massey", *Journal of African Civilizations,* I. Van Sertima, ed., 1982, 4(2): 63.
17 Massey, op. cit., passim.

the Pharaoh Zer ("Osiris"="*Asar*" or "*User*"), one of the kings of the 1st dynasty who was indubitably considered to have been a human avatar of Osiris by the Egyptians themselves.[18] Though Osiris was a deity who long pre-existed the historical Zer, it appears that Zer came to personify in human terms the god Osiris on earth. Thus the legend of Osiris being once a pharaoh of Egypt, as represented by Plutarch, might actually have had some basis in historical fact. With Buddha, a similar process can be seen. There were seven divine Buddhas prior to the historical Gautama, and the worship of Buddha reaches back into Indian proto-history when he was the god of the Black Dravidians of the Indus Valley city-states.[19] The historical Gautama by his life, deeds, and teachings became the incarnation of the eighth Buddha. The pre-extant Buddha mythology descended upon the figure of the historical Buddha, who was Gautama. Parenthetically, it might be mentioned that there are parallels elsewhere in Africa. Among the Yoruba, the worship of Shango revolves around a figure who was the first king of the kingdom of Oyo. This king evolved into the orisha of lightning and thunder, so that he is both man and god. Thus the process by which an extraordinary individual becomes the human avatar of a preexisting deity is well-attested throughout history. In the case of Imhotep, we see one of the earliest examples in which there is a merging of an historical man and a pre-extant deity.

18 Budge, E. A. W., *A History of Egypt,* Oosterhout N.B.: Anthropological Publications, vol. 1, 1968, pp. 20, 181.
19 See Higgins, G.,*Anacalypsis,* New Hyde Park: University Press, vol. 1, 1965, p. 53.

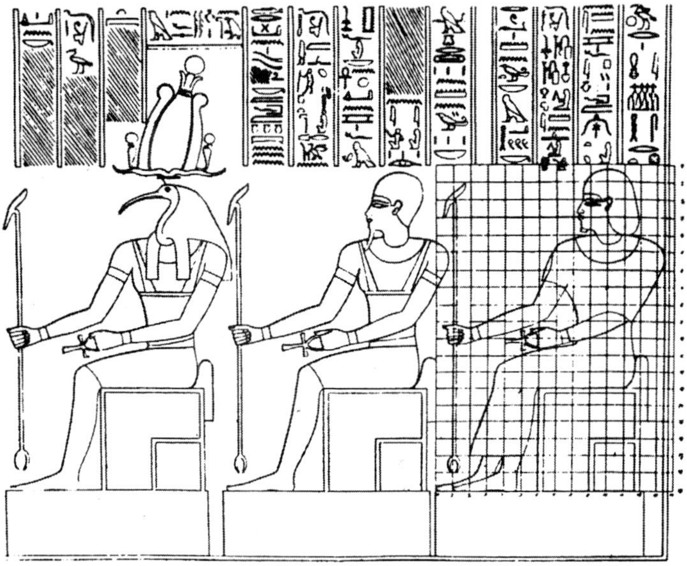

Figure 3
Thoth-Imhotep, and Amen-Hotep, son of Hapu.

Imhotep The God

As he came to be regarded as a deity, Imhotep was considered the "son of Ptah." In the process superseding the earliest form of the son of Ptah, Nefer-Tem, whose name means "the child Atum," shows a clear connection between the mythos of Ptah and that of Atum-Ra of Heliopolis. Massey maintains that Atum is first a son of Ptah prior to becoming a supreme deity in his own right:

> That son of Ptah was Turn or Atum ... and one of Atum's names or titles is Iu the coming son, or Iu-em-hetep, he who comes with peace.[20]

20 Massey, op. cit., p. 434.

The word "ptah" means "to open" which in this sense really means to "carve out, excavate, sculpt," etc. He is sometimes represented as a Twa with a scarab, the symbol of the god Khepera, on his crown. Kheper, the scarab, was a form of the creator as "the molder" because the scarab—also known as the Nile beetle—molds a ball of dung into which it deposits its eggs. It then rolls the ball of dung along the banks of the Nile and buries it in a small hole, where the ball containing the eggs remains until the Nile flood has subsided. After the period of incubation, the winged scarabs fly up out of the mud, providing a ready image of that which creates itself or resurrects itself out of the "primal ooze". Ptah as the "opener" and as the "molder" in his Khepera-form becomes one of the earliest images of the force of creation and he is represented in Egyptian iconography as a potter shaping and molding the World Egg on the potter's wheel. He is related to the Nubian ram-god Khnum who is represented as molding human beings out of clay on the potter's wheel. Under these circumstances, Imhotep's connection to Khnum in the Legend of the Seven Years' Famine becomes more intelligible. Ptah is pre-eminently the divine metallurgist, blacksmith, mason, and architect, attributes that he shares with Imhotep. Ptah was often represented as a Twa or a dwarf because these people were thought to know all the secrets of mining and metals.

E. A. Wallis Budge describes the godhood of Imhotep as follows:

> I-em-hetep was the god who sent sleep to those who were suffering and in pain, and those who were afflicted with any kind of disease formed his special charge; he was the good physician of both gods and men, and he healed the bodies

> of mortals during life, and superintended the arrangements for the preservation of the same after death.[21]

In this aspect, Imhotep is the bringer of peace and plenty, food and water, rest and succour:

> Iu-em-hetep, as is indicated by the name, comes to bring peace and goodwill to earth as conqueror of drought, dearth, and darkness.[22]

As we have seen, he is the wise and compassionate teacher, whose highest teachings were communicated orally, making him a personification of the Word or Logos.

> The expounder of the mysteries... was the Egyptian Jesus... as Iu-em-hetep, the prince of peace, and prototype of the Hebrew Solomon... The Egyptian Jesus was equally the Egyptian Solomon, the youthful sage, as sayer and teacher of the oral wisdom.[23]

In a sense then, Imhotep, famous for his wise sayings and proverbial wisdom, is recapitulated in the later figures of Solomon and Jesus, both revered for their oral wisdom teachings.

There were several temples dedicated to Imhotep that were built after the 6th century. The most famous of these was the temple of Imhotep in Memphis which in classical times was called "the Asclepeion". As we have noted earlier, it was so famous as a centre of healing and medical knowledge that many important post-Hippocratic Greek physicians, including Galen, The-

21 Budge, E. A. W., *Gods of the Egyptians,* New York: Dover Publications, vol. 1, 1969, p. 523.
22 Massey, op. cit., p. 418.
23 Ibid., p. 500.

ophrastus, and Dioscorides studied there.[24] It was located close to another famous healing temple, the Serapeum, dedicated to the god Serapis. Imhotep and Serapis were closely associated and this latter represented a late syncretization of Osiris and the divine Apis bull of Memphis who was a form of Ptah. This form of Osiris became paramount in the Hellenic and post-Hellenic period and was part of a trinity that included Isis and the Child Horus. The Romans identified Serapis worship with that of Christianity because the rituals and ceremonials were exactly the same.[25] Another Asclepeion dedicated to Imhotep existed on the "Holy Island" of Philae in Egyptian Nubia and rivalled the one in Memphis as a place of healing pilgrimage. Other temples dedicated to Imhotep and Asclepios were situated at Ptolemais Hermiu, and also, it seems in the Fayum, west of the Nile.[26] Hurry gives a good description of the phenomenon of "incubation" or "temple sleep" utilized by afflicted persons in these healing temples to obtain cures. When all other measures had failed, the sick person would be sent to the temple of the healing god, in this case Imhotep, to offer sacrifices and perform certain rituals to induce the god to send a cure. If these appeals were successful,the god would appear to the suppliant at night in a dream and give specific instructions on how a cure might be obtained. There are at least two surviving stories which illustrate the phe-

24 See note 8.

25 Massey, op. cit., p. 756. In a famous letter to Servianus, the Emperor Hadrian asserted, "those who worship Serapis are likewise Christians; even those who style themselves the Bishops of Christ are devoted to Serapis". Diodorus relates that all worshippers were given the name Serapis at their death and resurrection showing that Serapis, as a form of Osiris, was a holotype of Christ.

26 See Wilkinson, J. G., *The Manners and Customs of the Ancient Egyptians,* London: John Murray, vol. 3, 1878, p. 205.

nomenon of cure by incubation: both revolve around infertility. In the first story, the wife of a prince of the blood, who had produced no male children, repaired to the temple of Imhotep in her extremity where the god appeared to her in a dream telling her how she might conceive a son. The outcome was successful and the son went on to become a famous wise man. In this instance, the lady's infertility seemed only related to her capacity to bear a male child whereas in the second story, also involving a high-born woman, the sterility was absolute. Nonetheless, during the night in Imhotep's temple, the god appeared to her and provided her with instructions that would result in the birth of the son. In this case, the husband, a high priest, was required to carry out extensive works of renovation at a neglected sanctuary of Imhotep. This being done, a son was duly born and was named after Imhotep. It was commonplace in these cases for the child—born through the benign intervention of the god—to be dedicated to his service and we might presume that this is in fact what happened in the two stories related here. The Greeks too were well-acquainted with incubation and, as expected, it was the temple of Asclepios—Imhotep in his Greek form—that the suppliant visited to obtain cures. Robert Graves describes

> ... numerous oracles of Asclepius, where the sick flock for consultation and for cure, and are told the remedy in their dreams after a fast.[27]

If traditional healing in modern Africa offers any parallel, incubation served an additional function, for African traditional healers today insist that many of their remedies come to them in

27 Graves, R., *The Greek Myths*, New York:PenguinBooks, vol. 1, 1977,p. 179.

dreams, usually from a tutelary deity.[28] There is no reason not to believe that the priest-physicians attached to the House of Imhotep experienced something similar.

By mid-classical times, the worship of Imhotep had attained wide prominence. Temples, inscriptions, and bas-reliefs dedicated to him could be found throughout Egypt; moreover he had acquired membership in the important pantheons in Memphis, Philae, and Thebes.[29] In Nubia, his worship was as widespread as it was in Egypt, if the reliefs and inscriptions in that country are any indication. He is found in Meroe associated with the kings and rulers of that important city state. Moreover, his worship is not unknown among the Romans: at least two Roman emperors, Tiberius and Augustus, are represented in Egyptian temple reliefs doing him homage.

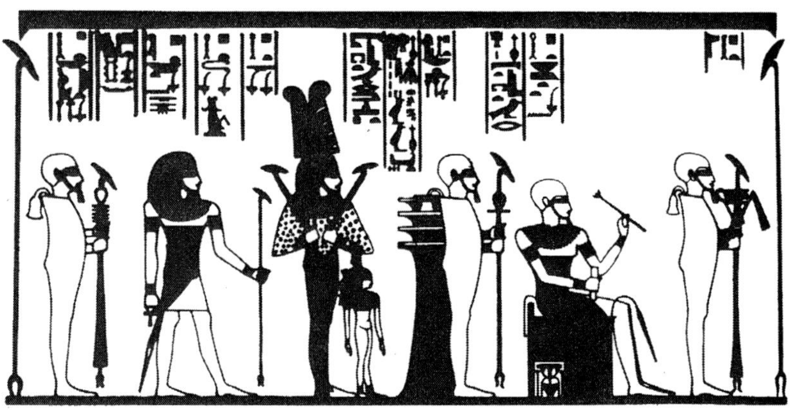

Figure 4

Various manifestations of Ptah, father of Imhotep.

28 Finch, Charles, *A knowledge, attitudes, and practices survey of traditional healers in Fatick, Senegal:* Final report, USAID Grant #685-0281-G00-1254-00, 1992, p.10

29 See Hurry, op. cit., pp. 62–144.

Imhotep and Asclepios

We have had cause to refer repeatedly to the identity of Imhotep and Asclepios and for this reason it is worth examining more closely the figure of Asclepios himself as the pre-eminent Greek god of healing. According to classical sources[30] Asclepios was the son of Apollo and a mortal princess Coronis, i.e., "the crow." Among the Greeks, the crow was an oracular bird and it had a similar connotation among the Egyptians though it was associated with the god Set. His mother, Coronis, died while carrying him and on her funeral pyre, Asclepios was cut from her womb by the god Hermes—Thoth in Greek form—at the command of Apollo. Asclepios was placed in the tutelage of Cheiron, the centaur, and became extraordinarily proficient in surgery and the healing powers of drugs and plants. For this reason he was referred to as the founder of medicine. He became so skilled in the healing art that he divined the secret of raising the dead to life. After restoring four dead heroes to life, he incurred the wrath of Hades who complained to Zeus that Asclepios was robbing him of his rightful subjects. For this impious presumption, Zeus struck Asclepios dead with a thunderbolt. His father Apollo whereupon killed the cyclopes, renowned as masons and metalworkers, for having forged the thunderbolts of Zeus. Later, Zeus repented of his rash action and restored Asclepios to life as a deity of medicine. The symbol of Asclepios was the serpent and the staff—derived from the caduceus of Hermes—and when the early Romans wished to establish the worship of Asclepios in

30 For a complete survey of all of the classical references to Asclepios, see Graves, op. cit., pp. 173–8.

their own lands, Epidauros, the site of an important Asclepeion, sent them an avatar of the god in the form of a snake.[31]

The mythic history of Asclepios, with his theogamy, commends several things to our attention. Though ostensibly the son of Apollo, Asclepios is in fact removed from his mother's womb by Hermes, establishing a connection that echoes the fact that Imhotep was considered to be "the image of Thoth",[32] whom the Greeks called Hermes. The mother of Asclepios, "Coronis the Crow", by virtue of her name would have been an oracle priestess and we know that the temples of Asclepios were, in effect, healing oracles. Asclepios is considered, like Imhotep, a mortal son of a divine father who becomes translated into a deity of healing. The somewhat tangential part that the cyclopes play in the myth still echoes the fact that they, like Imhotep and his divine father Ptah, are masons, metalworkers, and builders. Finally, the snake twined around the staff is a motif originally associated with Thoth, the first healing god of the Egyptian pantheon. The original Greek god of healing, Hermes, takes it directly from him. The snake was a potent symbol of renewal and resurrection because of its ability to slough old skin for new. This made it one of the earliest healing types. All things considered, it is no wonder that the Greeks made Asclepios their Imhotep: there was a pronounced reverence among them for things Egyptian and all of their important healing symbols were prefigured in Egypt. Their names were used interchangeably so ubiquitously that in the Greek mind they were one and same.

31 Majno, op. cit., p. 339.
32 See Hurry, op. cit., pp. 60, 66.

The Hermetic Imhotep

Some mention must be made of Imhotep in the Hermetic or "Trismegistic" literature. The Hermetic corpus represented a fusion of ancient Egyptian thought and Greek philosophy, with the Egyptian elements clearly predominating. It was an esoteric school—allied to and interacting with similar schools such as Gnosticism—that exerted a powerful if sub-rosa influence on early Christianity, and later Medieval thought. Alchemy and Astrology were considered branches of the Hermetic science, and later Freemasonry and Rosicrucianism drew deeply from Hermetic currents. Though anathemized by orthodox Christianity, it is a remarkable fact that the great scientists, philosophers, statesmen, and artists of the Western world were devotees of the various branches of the Hermetic art. Roger Bacon and Paracelcus were alchemists, Copernicus and Newton were astrologers, Washington, Mozart, Napoleon, and Kipling were Freemasons. The paragon of the Hermetic work was Hermes Trismegistus, Hermes the "Thrice-Greatest", who was considered the quintessential Master of all knowledge and wisdom. His three important disciples are Asclepios, Tat, and Ammon. All of these figures represent anthropomorphized Egyptian deities: Asclepios is of course Imouthes/Imhotep, Tat is Thoth, and Ammon is the Theban Amen. Other Egyptian deities figure prominently in the Hermetic mythos. These are Anubis, Khnum, here called Chnum, and Lady Isis. In its surviving fragments, Hermetic philosophy unfolds in a series of Socratic-like discourses between the Master Hermes and his disciples. In this framework, Asclepius-Imhotep carries the titles of "king" and "divine saviour;"[33] and he comes

33 Mead, G. R. S., *Thrice Greatest Hermes,* London: John M. Watkins, vol. 1949, p. 469.

forward in the hermetic opus as the one disciple who is already well-schooled in philosophy. G. R. S. Mead says

> Tat and Asclepius share a common instruction—Asclepius appearing as the older and riper scholar.[34]

Tat, however, is the "St. John" of the three disciples, the one who has Hermes' highest favour and the one who will carry on the authentic teaching. It must be remembered that Tat—being the personification of Thoth—is but an aspect of Hermes himself which would account for his favoured position. We have noted

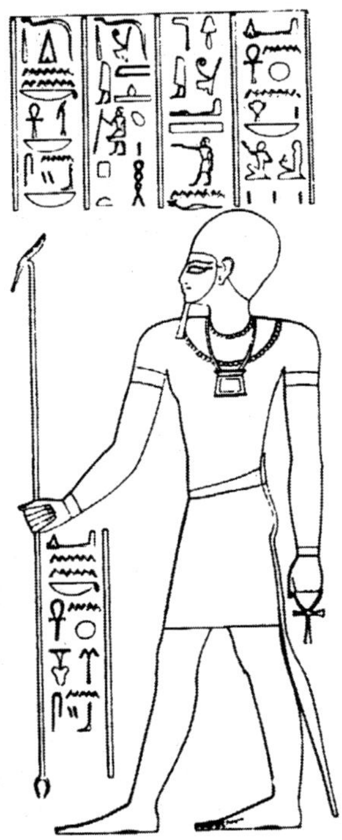

Figure 5a
Imhotep, the god, Bringer of Peace and Plenty.

34 Ibid., p. 471.

earlier how Imhotep was called "the image of Thoth", and we see how—as one of the three disciples of Trismegistus—this is reflected in Hermetic tradition. Hermetic tradition further characterizes him as a "master mason, inventor of poetry, healer, and master astrologer",[35] in effect, carrying him and his attributes forward from his place in the pantheons of old Egypt.

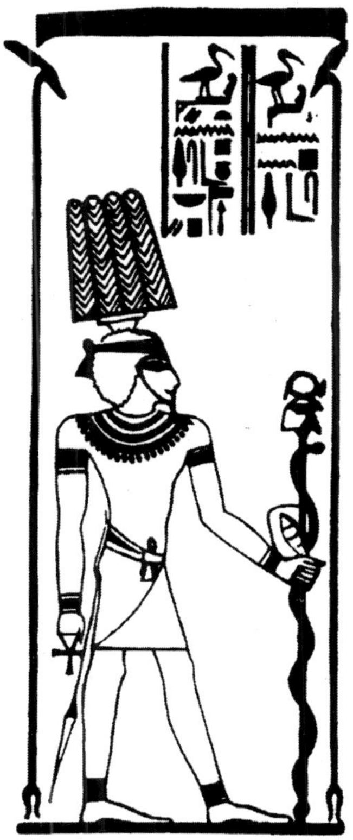

Figure 5b
Thoth, god of medicine with the Caduceus in his hand.

35 Ibid., pp. 464–76; see also Hurry, op. cit., pp. 27, 30, 36, 41.

Epilogue

Greek thought and philosophy, both esoteric and exoteric, was lifted bodily out of the Egyptian world system, and no one figured more prominently in this process than Imhotep as man, god, sage, and symbol. Though we possess mere fragments of his true personal history, he still comes through as a man of

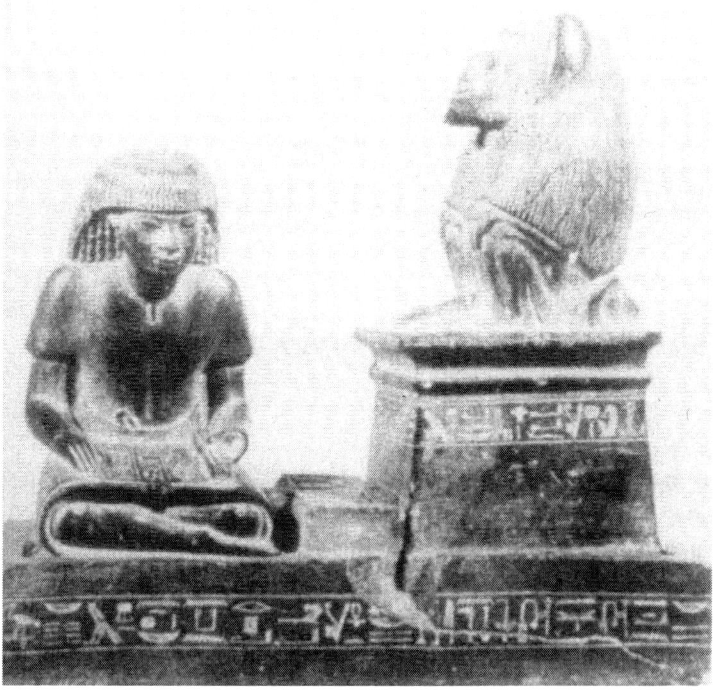

Figure 6
Thoth-Hermes, master of learning in his form as cynocephalicape, seen here dictating to a scribe.

extraordinary capacity. He seems to have achieved a perfect synthesis of mind, intellect, and soul—so much so that men thought they saw in him the spark of divinity. The centuries, rather than dimming this spark in men's minds, seemed to have fanned it to a bright flame. As a consequence, Imhotep the man became Imhotep the god. Massey considered him the prototype of the Saviour and this is corroborated in Hermetic tradition. As physician, builder, and sage, he was the archetype of the Great Man.

CHAPTER THREE

Science and Symbol in Egyptian Medicine

In our own time, we are accustomed to attributing the beginnings of scientific medicine to the Greek physician Hippocrates who lived in the 5th century B.C. It is said that the foundations of a purely clinical approach to illness exemplified by techniques of history-taking, examination, diagnosis, prognosis, and empirical therapy begins with Hippocrates and his School, reaching its greatest development in classical times with Galen. Thus Hippocrates has been styled the "Father of Medicine" and physicians all over the world take the semi-sacred Hippocratic Oath upon completion of their medical studies. But who was Hippocrates really? He has exercised an immense influence on medicine for nearly 25 centuries and we would think that he was a clear-cut historical figure. However, on closer inspection, he is rather dim and shadowy. We know that he was born on the island of Cos, the descendant of a line of priests of Asclepios, that he became a physician of renown, and that he was revered enough as a physician that eventually an entire school sprung up around his teachings. But we don't know much more than that:

> Practically nothing is known of his life but many legends have sprung up about this great doctor and teacher.
>
> Even two hundred years after his death, no one knew anything definite about Hippocrates' life.[1]

Only a fraction of the large Hippocratic written corpus can be directly attributed to him and he cannot even claim authorship of the fabled Hippocratic Oath. In all fairness to him, however, he never gave himself the title "Father of Medicine" nor is there any reason to doubt that he was a physician of unusual gifts. Moreover, it becomes glaringly evident through a study of the Egyptian medical papyri that Hippocrates and his followers drew heavily upon the theory and practice of ancient Egyptian medicine.[2] So heavy was this indebtedness that had Hippocrates ever had the question of priority put to him he might well have echoed the dictum of Homer who in the *Odyssey* stated, "In medical knowledge, Egypt leaves the rest of the world behind." In fact in some ways, Hippocrates had not even advanced as far as the ancient Egyptians before him. He never mentions pulse-taking and considered the brain to have been a gland.[3] To cite but two examples in therapeutics, the Hippocratic methods of setting clavicular fractures and reducing a dislocated mandible are almost exactly as described in the Edwin Smith Papyrus.[4] There are many more examples that could be cited of the pronounced similarity of important facets of Hippocratic medicine to ancient Egyptian medicine and, based on the historically verifiable pattern of cul-

1 Bogdonoff, M.D., et al, editors, "Introduction" to *The Aphorisms of Hippocrates,* Birmingham, The Classics of Medicine Library, 1982, p. 3.

2 Ghalioungui, P., *The House of Life: Magic and Medical Science in Ancient Egypt,* Amsterdam, B. M., Israel, 1973, p. 31.

3 Ibid., p. 41.

4 Ibid., p. 42.

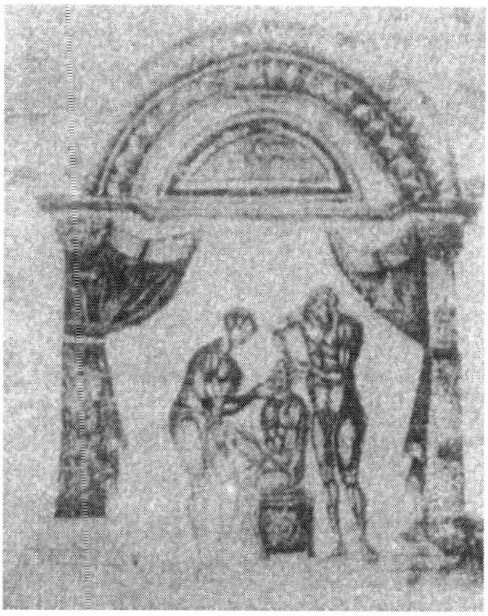

Figure 1
Hippocratic method for reducing a dislocation of the jaw, first described in the Edwin Smith papyrus.

tural borrowing of Greece from Egypt, this indicates that much of Hippocratic medicine was Egyptian medicine in Greek form.

This idea is given greater weight when we examine the Alexandrian school of Greek medicine, of whom Galen was the greatest exponent. In fact, the Alexandrian period represents the Golden Age of Greek Medicine in which startling discoveries in anatomy and physiology were made. This rather sudden efflorescence of Greek medicine at Alexandria can be attributed to one major cause: the collection of all available Egyptian scientific papyri by the early Ptolemies under the roof of the Library of Alexandria. This justly-famous library at its height contained over 700,000 volumes and made the city the intellectual centre of the classical world. The scientific renaissance of the Alexandrian period was therefore due to the Greek world's unlimited access to the learning of ancient Egypt. The famous "discoveries" by the Greek scientists of that time were, for the most part, "re-discoveries" of ancient Egyptian learning and thought. Herophilus, an Alexandrian Greek of the 4th century B.C., is ordinarily credited with the discovery of the diagnostic applications of pulse-taking; though we now know that this was described in both the Ebers and Smith medical papyri 35 centuries before his time. It seems likely that Herophilus had access to the ancient Egyptian *Book of the Heart and Vessels,* the same source of information used by the ancient Egyptian authors of the Ebers and Smith papyri. Moreover, Herophilus and his Alexandrian contemporary, Erasistratus, are usually credited with first delineating the relations between the peripheral nerves and the central nervous system. But a modern medical historian says about the Edwin Smith Papyrus:

> It is difficult to escape the conclusion that the author clearly realized the relationship between the nervous system and voluntary movements and the fact that the side and localization of the paralysis depend on the situation of the nervous lesion.[5]

He goes on to say,

> It is, therefore, interesting to point out again that these two learned physicians (Herophilus and Erasistratus) practiced in Alexandria in Egypt... while five centuries later Greek physicians were still visiting Egypt to consult the library at Memphis.[6]

5 Ibid., pp. 40–41.
6 Ibid.

Galen, himself, though a member of the Hippocratic School, spent many years in Alexandria furthering his medical education. Nor did Galen and his physician contemporaries limit themselves to Alexandria, also traveling to the famous healing temples and libraries of Sais and Memphis in search of medical knowledge. It is therefore in vain that we look to Greece for the origins of modern medicine; we can only do so in ancient Egypt, the teacher of the Greeks.

In Chapter 1, the present author provided an introduction to an African medical science that began in Egypt but continued its development, in often remarkable ways, elsewhere in Africa.[7] In this chapter we will examine Egyptian medical science more closely, through the agency of the Edwin Smith Papyrus, to understand better its impact on the history of medicine.

Before proceeding with a discussion of Egyptian medicine, a short space must be devoted to the question of Egyptian chronology. Since the beginning of Egyptology as a scholarly discipline, there have been running debates about Egyptian chronology which, broadly speaking, are divided into two camps: the "long" chonology vs. the "short" chronology. The long chronology, propounded by scholars such as Lepsius, Petrie, and Budge, dates the beginning of the Egyptian dynastic period—that is the unification of the Two Lands under Menes—somewhere between 5,000 and 4,000 B.C. This was the dominant view until the early part of this century when Meyer proposed a date of 3400 B.C. for the beginning of the 1st dynasty. Since then Egyptologists have, by convention, adopted modifications of Meyer's scheme

7 Finch, C., "The African Background of Medical Science", *Blacks in Science: Ancient and Modern,* I. Van Sertima, editor, New Brunswick: *Journal of African Civilizations,* Ltd., 1983, pp. 148–55.

so that now the dominant opinion dates the beginning of Egyptian history around 3100 B.C. The argument turns around three important elements used to reconstruct Egyptian chronology: 1) the history of Manetho which divides Egyptian history into 30 dynasties of 330 kings, covering a space of more than 5,000 years, 2) surviving fragments of king lists that appear on the Turin Papyrus, the Palermo Stone, etc., and 3) the 1460-year Sothic cycle which is determined by the gradual backward slippage of the Egyptian civil year of 365 days in relation to the Sothic year of 365¼ days. This Sothic year of 365 ¼ days was determined by the heliacal rising of the star Sirius, the brightest of the stars seen from Earth, coincident with the beginning of the annual Nile Flood which marked the beginning of the Egyptian New Year. Because there is a discrepancy of ¼ day between the two years, it takes 1460 years (1460 x ¼ = 365) for the two calendars to coincide again. The short chronology rests on two assumptions: 1) a revision of Manetho in which numerous dynasties in the two Intermediate Periods are conflated, thereby reducing the length of time attested to by Manetho by 2,000 years and 2) that the Egyptians did *not* begin using the Sothic year until the beginning of a new cycle about 2780 B.C. The first rationale is dubious and the second is simply inadmissable. Surviving inscriptions from the 1st dynasty, that is *prior* to 2780 B.C., refer to the relationship between the heliacal rising of Sirius, the beginning of the flood, and the New Year.[8] This means that the Egyptians *had* to have known of the Sothic cycle before 2780 B.C. which, by referring to the date of the beginning of the previous cycle, goes

8 See Lamy, *L., Egyptian Mysteries,* New York: Crossroad, 1981, p. 6, for a reproduction of an ivory tablet from the 1st dynasty on which is inscribed the words "Sirius, Opener of the Year, Inundation 1".

back to 4240 B.C., the first identifiable calendar date in history. The existence of a highly sophisticated calendar at such a remote period means that there had to have been a civilization in place advanced enough to have acquired and recorded the astronomical knowledge necessary for the creation of such a calendar. The lopping off of great segments of time from Manetho's history, in the scheme of the short chronology, is therefore not entirely defensible. There is reason to believe, after Budge, that the first dynasty of Menes actually begins around 4400 B.C.—or shortly thereafter—instead of the received date of 3100 B.C., pushing Egyptian history back 1200 years or so.

What does this have to do with our subject? Breasted, the translator and commentator of the Edwin Smith Papyrus, has demonstrated by linguistic analysis that the extant manuscript, though written during the 18th dynasty (circa 1500 B.C.), is actually a late copy of an original first produced early in the Old Kingdom, perhaps as early as the 1st Dynasty. But if we date the beginning of the Old Kingdom sometime between 4400–4200 B.C., i.e., close to the earliest calendar date, then the Edwin Smith Papyrus reflects medical knowledge that existed in northeast Africa 6,000 years ago. Moreover, it is a mature scientific document, the culmination of a long period of anterior development. This means that the true beginnings of what we think of as scientific medicine are so remote as to be lost to the gaze of history.

The level of medical science revealed in the Edwin Smith Papyrus makes it the most remarkable medical document to survive from antiquity. The present translation is the fruit of the marvelous scholarship of James Henry Breasted who, after 10 years of work, published his version in 1930. Breasted included an extensive commentary and was immensely aided in his labors by physician colleagues. His translation has stood the test of time and remains the standard one for the Edwin Smith Papyrus.

It is in Egypt, as exemplified by the Edwin Smith Papyrus, that the first anatomical descriptions appear in a systematic way. More than two hundred different anatomical parts have been described in the extant Egyptian medical literature.[9] Many of these terms appear in the Edwin Smith Papyrus. Breasted is entirely correct when he asserts that one reason why this document is so valuable is that it preserves for us a record of a scientific vocabulary in evolution. The first treatise writer(s) not only inherited, but modified and created terms to describe the anatomy and pathological conditions, giving us a medical vocabulary that is 6,000 years old. The language of these early medical terms was very archaic, so that by the time the redaction of the original manuscript occurred around 1500 B.C., it was necessary for the editor to append glosses to explain the otherwise impenetrable meanings.

In this chapter, the author provides lists and illustrations depicting the various anatomical and medical terms gleaned from the surviving medical papyri.[10] It is to be noted that the anatomical terms derived from the Edwin Smith Papyrus focus almost exclusively on the skeletal and soft tissue parts of the head and neck. It was originally a treatise dealing systematically with traumatic injuries from the head down. Unfortunately, the 18th dynasty copyist broke off after the 48th case, so that only the upper third of the body, i.e., the head and neck, were covered in

9 Ghalioungui, op. cit., p. 48.

10 Sec Leca, A. P., *La Médecine Egyptienne,* Paris: Les Editions Roger DaCosta, 1983 and Schwaller de Lubicz, R. A., *Le Temple De L'Homme,* Volume 1, Paris: Caracteres, 1960 for lists of Egyptian medical and anatomical terms.

this edition. Though the original was undoubtedly a complete manual of traumatic surgery, the Edwin Smith Papyrus represents only one-third of it.

Breasted is of the opinion that the original author was probably a military surgeon since the majority of the cases involve the kind of trauma most likely sustained in combat. Other medical historians are of the opinion that the original compiler of this surgical manual actually drew upon his experiences treating traumatic injuries incurred during the construction of the Great Pyramid.[11] Yet the traumatic injuries described in the Edwin Smith Papyrus are much more easily reconciled to the assumption that they were received in combat. The nature and location of the wounds and injuries depicted are best understood as being delivered by hand-held weapons. According to Breasted, the original author was a battlefield surgeon who wrote this treatise as a capstone to a career full of varied surgical experience in the field. This is undoubtedly true as far as it goes, but the Edwin Smith Papyrus conveys the distinct impression that the author was also drawing upon a reservoir of past knowledge. It is hard not to believe that, while writing this manual, he immersed himself in the medical literature written by his predecessors and amplified this "book" research with his own direct experience. The author does actually cite *The Book of What Pertains to the Embalmer* and *The Book of What Pertains to His Wounds* as references.[12] Our author was

11 Ghalioungui, op. cit., p. 44.

12 Breasted, J. H., *The Edwin Smith Papyrus,* Birmingham: The Classics of Medicine Library, 1984, pp 434, 446. The titles that the ancient author refers to in Breasted's translation are rendered respectively as "Treatise on What Pertains to His Wounds" and "Treatise on What Pertains to the Embalmer".

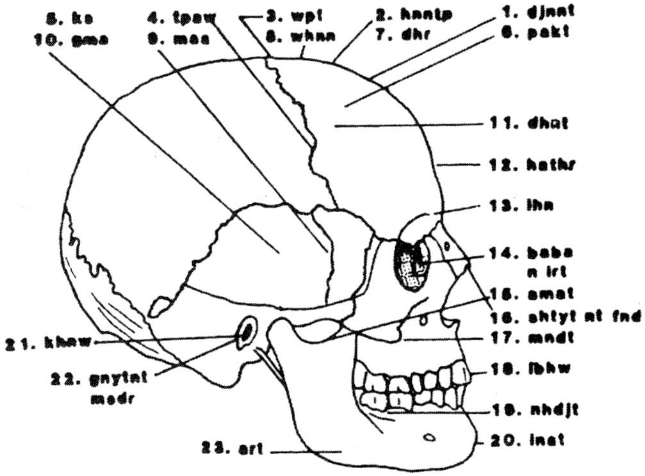

Figure 2
*Some Anatomical Terms of the Cranium**

Egyptian	*English*	*Egyptian*	*English*
1. djnnt	cranium	13. ihn	superciliary arch (eyebrow)
2. hn n tp	cranial vault	14. baba n irt	orbit
3. wpt	vertex	15. amât	mandibular notch
4. tpaw	cranial suture	16. shtyt nt fnd	bony nasal chamber
5. ks	bone	17. mndt	cheek bone
6. pakt	cranial bone	18. ibhw	teeth
7. dhr	suture membrane	19. nhdjt	molars (?)
8. whnn	bregma*	20. inât	chin
9. maâ	temporal region	21. khnw	internal auditory canal
10. gma	temporal bone	22. gnyt nt msdjr	external auditory canal
11. dhnt	frontal bone		
12. hat hr	forehead	23. ârt	body of the mandible

* junction of coronal & sagittal sutures

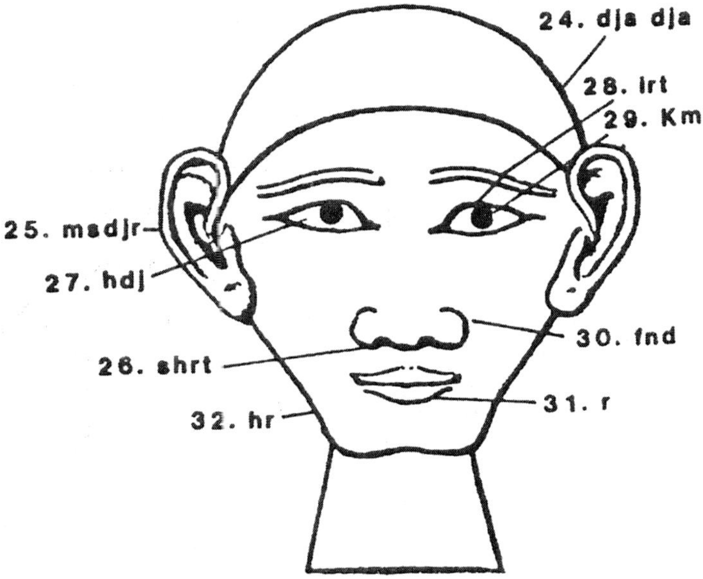

Figure 3
Some Anatomical Terms of the Face

Egyptian	*English*
24. djadja	head (entire)
25. msdjr	ear
26. shrt	nostril
27. hdj	sclera (white of the eye)
28. irt	eye
29. km	pupil ("black" of the eye)
30. fnd	nose
31. r	mouth
32. hr	face

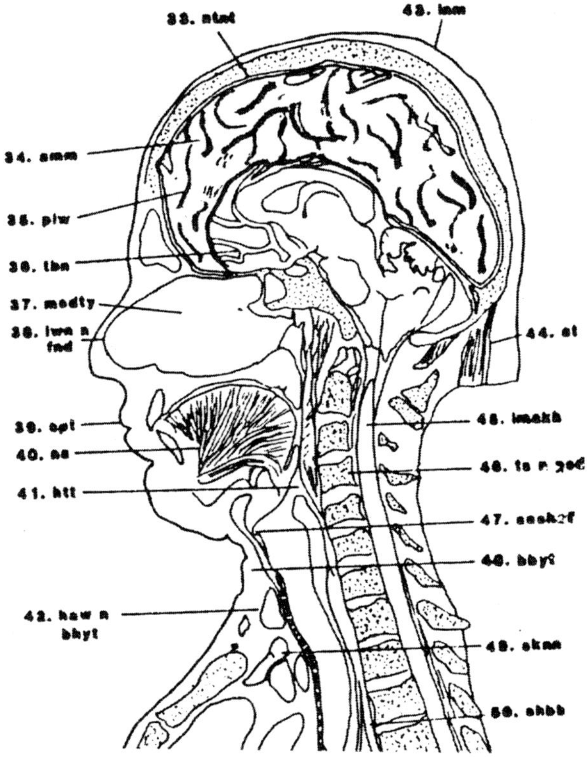

Figure 4

Some Soft Tissue Terms of the Head & Neck

Egyptian	*English*	*Egyptian*	*English*
33. ntnt	meninges	42. hâw n bbyt	thyroid(?)
34. âmm	cerebrum, brain	43. inm	skin
35. piw	convolutions (of brain)	44. ât	muscle
36. tbn	brain	45. imakh	spinal cord
37. msdty	nasal fossa	46. ts n psd	dorsal (cervical) vertebra
38. iwn n fnd	nasal cartilage	47. sashat	larynx
39. spt	lip	48. bbyt	supra-clavicular region
40. ns	tongue	49. sknn	thymus(?)
41. htt	pharynx	50. shbb	esophagus

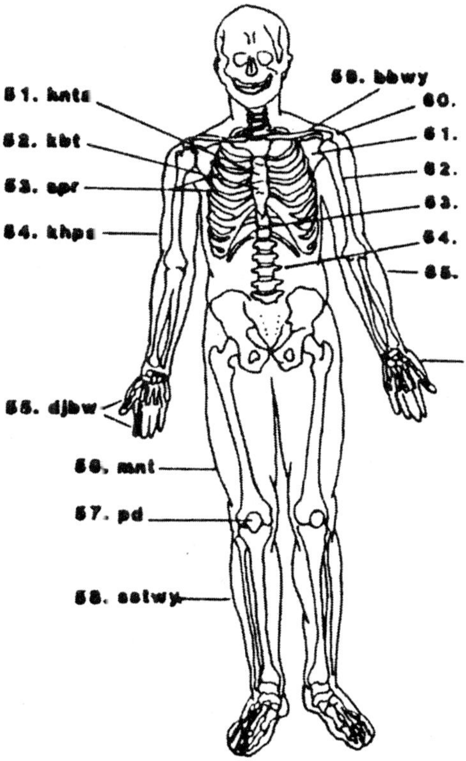

Figure 5

Some Anatomical Terms of the Skeleton

Egyptian	*English*	*Egyptian*	*English*
51. hnta	manubrium	59. bbwy	clavicles
52. kbt	sternum	60. rmn	shoulder
53. spr	ribs	61. mshâkt	scapula
54. khps	arm	62. gb	humerus
55. djbw	fingers	63. psd	back
56. mnt	thigh	64. djs n psd	thoracic vertibra
57. pd	patella	65. â	forearm
58. sstwy	calves	66. djrt	hand

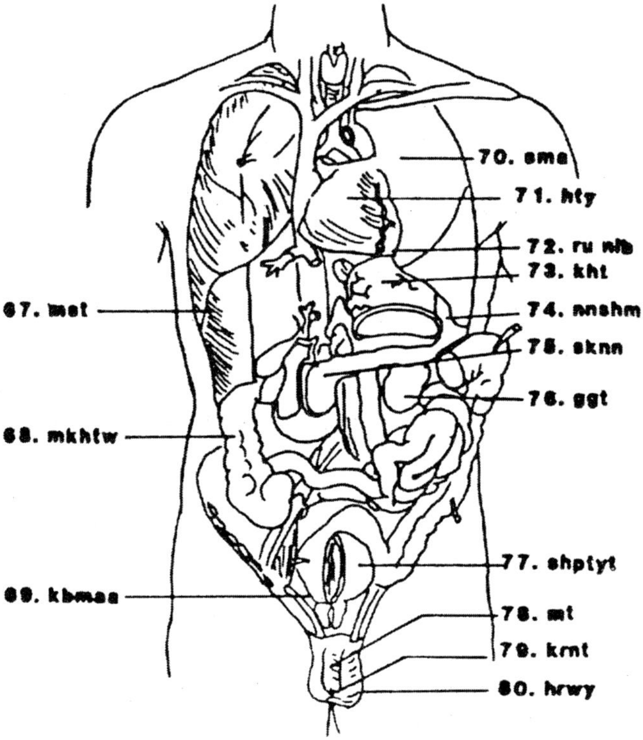

Figure 6
*Some Anatomical Terms of the Viscera**

Egyptian	*English*	*Egyptian*	*English*
67. mst	liver	74. nnshm	spleen
68. mkhtw	intestine	75. sknn	pancreas
69. kbmaâ	rectum	76. ggt	kidney
70. sma	lung	77. shptyt	bladder
71. hty	heart (pericardium)	78. mt	phallus
72. ru n ib	cardia	79. krnt	prepuce
73. kht	stomach	80. hrwy	testicle

*Figure shows overlying organs cut away to reveal interior organs.

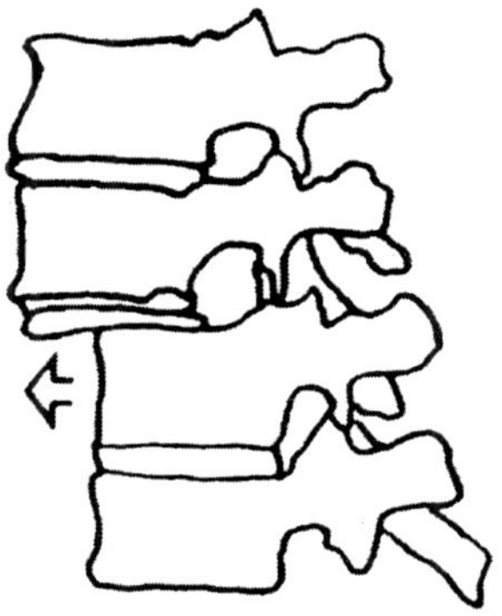

Figure 7
Vertebral Dislocation (See Case 31)

unquestionably a brilliant scholar, clinician, and writer, unifying these gifts to a degree rare in any age.

Of the more than 200 anatomical terms identified in the Egyptian medical literature, nearly 100 are found in the Edwin Smith Papyrus. However, this was a surgical treatise, and though filled with anatomical terms, we cannot assume that it or any of the other surviving medical papyri necessarily exhaust Egyptian anatomical terminology or contain the sum total of Egyptian anatomical knowledge. In our own time, only a textbook of anatomy would contain all of the thousands of anatomical terms used in modern medicine. Manetho informs us that Athothis, the second pharaoh of the 1st dynasty, was a physician who wrote a textbook of anatomy. It is tempting to speculate that such a treatise—which was contemporaneous with the Edwin Smith Papyrus—would have contained many more terms than the ones that have survived to the present. Even more of the true extent of Egyptian anatomical knowledge would have been revealed had this textbook survived. Reading through the Edwin Smith

Papyrus there is the sense that the Egyptians had more knowledge of anatomy and surgery than we are accustomed to giving them credit for. Moreover, we assume that whatever anatomical knowledge they did come by was serendipitously acquired from the purely ritualistic dissections that accompanied the funerary ceremonies. We know that elsewhere in Africa, bodies were dissected on quasi-clinical grounds,[13] but nothing of the sort is documented in the literature of ancient Egypt prior to the Alexandrian period when the ban against clinical dissection was lifted by the Ptolemies. Yet in reading through the Edwin Smith Papyrus, one cannot escape the conclusion that the Egyptian priest-physicians either used the thousands of funerary dissections for scientific instruction or found a way to perform purely clinical dissections.

There is a body of opinion, now somewhat diminished, that assumes that the ancient Egyptians had no knowledge of the mental functions of the human brain. Probably this is due to the Egyptians' habit of locating the anatomical seat of the soul, conscience, and feeling in the heart. One of their reasons for doing so may be related to the keen sensitivity of the heart to mental and emotional states. The Egyptian word for "heart" in this usage is "ib". Today we still used terms such as "hard-hearted", "tender-hearted", or "heart-broken" to describe emotional states or character types. There is a new area of study called "neurocardiology" that describes an interplay between the brain and the heart. The heart is constantly modifying and modulating our body's response to stress and emotion through electric, pressure wave, hormonal, and electromagnetic—or energy—communication

13 See Finch, op. cit., p. 149.

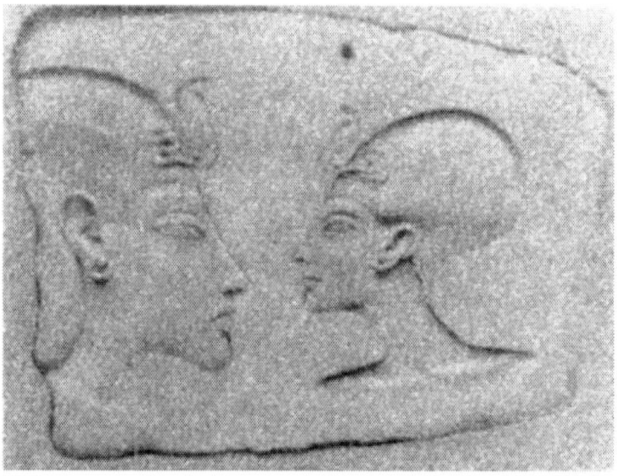

Figure 8
The head of the raised serpent is exactly level with the vertex on both crowns of this royal pair.

from the heart to the brain.[14] The ancient Egyptians may have known something that we are only recently discovering.

There is, however, simply no basis for assuming that the Egyptians did not know that the brain was the seat of all mental functioning. In fact the topmost part of the cranium, the vertex, is of tremendous importance in the pharaonic mythos. It supports the crown which is fronted by the raised uraeus serpent, the symbol of divine and royal power. This raised serpent is positioned in such a way that the very top of the serpent's head, as it juts out from the pharaoh's forehead, is exactly on a level with the vertex of the cranium. The body of this "cranial" serpent extends backward in a sinuous fashion exactly down the middle of the cranium, attaching to the circular band that surrounds the head. This body of the serpent effectively divides the cranium into two equal halves,

14 See *HeartMath® Institute*. J.A. Armour. and G.C. Kember, *Cardiac sensory neurons* in J.A. Armour and J.L. Ardell, editors, *Basic and Clinical Neurocardiology*, 2004, Oxford University Press: New York, pp. 79–117.

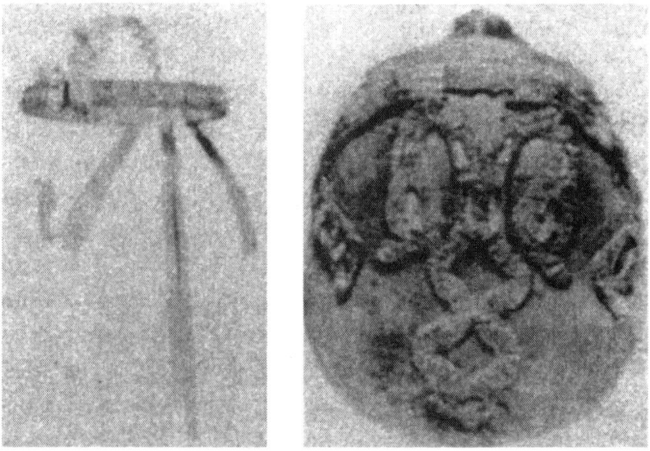

Figure 9a (left)
Uraeus Crown. The serpentine body recapitulates the sagittal suture of the cranium.
Figure 9b (right)
The mummified crown of Tutankhamen in which the double uraeus serpent conjoins the two hemispheres of the brain.

or hemispheres, and symbolically serves the same purpose as the sagittal suture of the cranium. This serpent is therefore emblematic of that which divides while it unifies. What is of further interest is that the Egyptian name for the cranial vertex is "wpt" which means "to open"; also "to discern" or "to judge", a clear reference to the cerebrum as the seat of judgement. But the symbolism inherent in the term "wpt" also signifies the "opening" of the higher cortical centres that corresponds to the "awakened" state, in this way identical to the rising of the Kundalini Serpent of Tantric Yoga that climbs from the base of the spine to the top of the head during the course of spiritual exercises. The opening of the transcendental eye of spiritual vision occurs when this serpent energy reaches the vertex. It is significant that among the ritual kings and traditional priests of Africa, their power is said to reside in their heads; even in the rural South of the United States, the successful Voodoo doctor is said to be "strong in his head".[15]

Another datum that refutes the opinion that the Egyptians were unaware of the thinking functions of the brain comes from a linguistic analysis of an Egyptian word for "cerebrum" which is "âmm". This word also means "to know" and "to understand", which defines, therefore, the anatomical cerebrum *and* its mental function.[16]

Scarab and Skull Crown
Symbolic Comparison

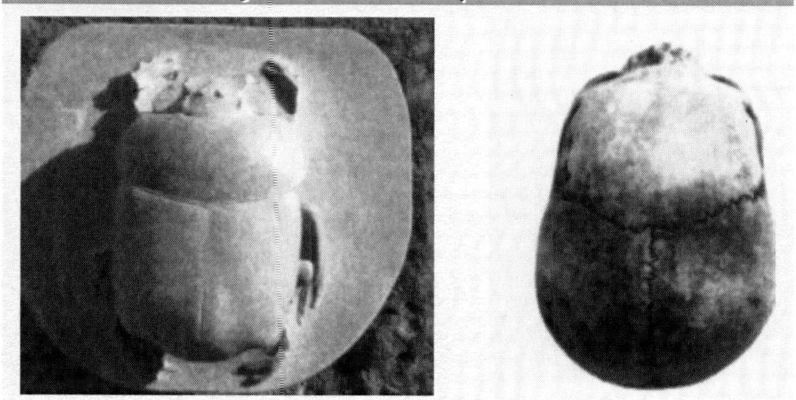

As revealed in the Edwin Smith Papyrus, the Egyptians not only designated the gross anatomy of the brain but also defined certain specific portions of it and their functions. One of their words for the temporal region of the skull was "maâ" and it is in the temporal region that the centres for hearing and speaking

15 Puckett, N. N., *The Magic and Folk Beliefs of the Southern Negro,* New York: Dover Publications, Inc., 1969, p. 189.

16 Budge, E. A. W., *An Egyptian Hieroglyphic Dictionary,* New York: Dover Publications, Inc., 1978, pp. 120–21.

are situated. Thus one of the Egyptian locutions for "to listen" was "to give the maâ" in the same way we might say "lend an ear".[17] This locution for "to listen" does not, therefore, refer to the anatomical ear but to the sites in the brain where sounds are processed to give hearing. This is but one indication in the Edwin Smith Papyrus that the ancient Egyptians had identified and localized this important cortical centre.

That the Egyptians had accurately mapped the internal anatomy of the head may be revealed in the anatomical phrase "wab n irt", which means literally "the root of the eye". According to Schwaller de Lubicz, this idea of "the root of the eye" related to the nourishing functions of the vessels and nerves (mtw) and conforms to an actual anatomical reality. He points out that as the optic nerve enters the posterior aspect of the eye, it contains in its sheath the retinal artery which in truth does "nourish" the posterior portion of the eye.[18] He further tells us,

> "Root of the eye" cannot signify the orbital cavity, but really does mean "root" which is designated by its determinative, a small plant. But the root is what nourishes the plant and it is therefore certain that the text, by "root", means to connote all of the nerve and blood channels...
>
> ...the authors of this old papyrus knew very well the internal anatomy of the cranium.[19]

One of the most salient anatomical descriptions in the Edwin Smith Papyrus is that of the brain along with its convolutions and meningeal covering. Though we will comment on the brain's gross anatomy later, it is worthwhile here to explore the

17 See Schwaller de Lubicz, op. cit., p. 568.
18 Ibid., p. 572.
19 Ibid., p. 573.

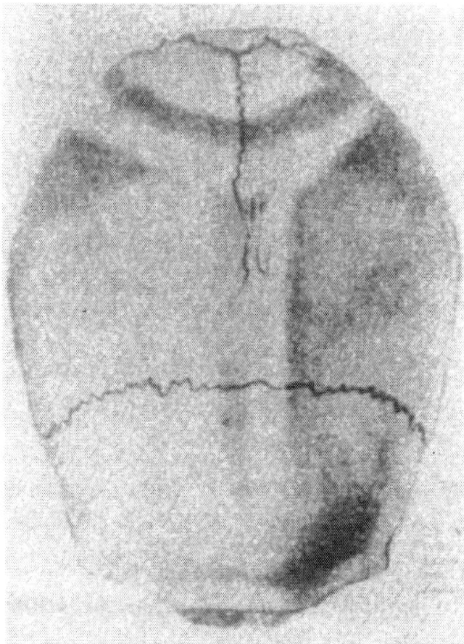

Figure 10
Cranial scar on a prehistoric female skull—the "opening" (cf. note para 24).

Egyptians' concept of the meninges and their function. The Latin name that we use for the meninges is "mater", meaning "mother", and they consist of three layers: 1) the dura mater ("hard mother"), the tough, fibrous, outer layer that is directly apposite to the interior of the bony cranium; 2) the pia mater ("soft mother"), the soft, pliable inner meningeal layer that adheres closely to the outer substance of the brain itself; 3) the arachnoid ("spider-like"), a fine, reticulated, web-like membrane situated between the outer layer of the dura mater and the inner layer of the pia mater. The Egyptian word for meninges is "netnet", suggesting by the doubling of the word "net", the apparent two-fold nature of the meninges on gross inspection.[20] This term "net" is quite interesting: it is the Egyptian word for "weaving" and for "water".[21] It is also the Egyptian name for Neith, the Virgin Mother goddess and the goddess of weaving, whose inscription on the entrance to her temple at Sais bore these words:

> I am all that has been, that is, or shall be. No mortal shall lift my veil.

The meninges symbolically are the woven "veil" which encloses the brain and spinal cord. The meninges also enclose the cerebrospinal fluid in which the entire brain and spinal cord structures are bathed, and we have seen how the root word "net" can also mean "water" or "fluid". Our Latin terminology "mater", or "mother", for the meninges is allusive to the most important aspect of Neith as one of the earliest Egyptian forms of the Great Mother. In this guise she is connected to water in her manifestation as the sky-goddess Nut, Mistress of the Celestial Waters. This simple root "net", by giving us in its duplicative form the Egyptian word for "meninges", contains an ensemble of meanings which resonate between the science and symbol of ancient Egypt.

The Egyptian word for cerebrospinal fluid—which bathes the brain and the spinal cord—is "nkh". We have already called attention to the special significance of our Latin terminology for the meninges, "mater" or "mother", and it should be no less interesting to us that the Egyptian word "nkh" can also signify "child" or "babe".[22] Taking the meninges, the cerebrospinal fluid, and

20 Ibid., p. 583. In gross appearance, the meninges are a two-fold membrane; the third layer of the meninges, the arachnoid, is not readily observable on external inspection because it is "sandwiched" between the dura mater and the pia mater.

21 See Budge, op. cit., pp. 399–400.

22 Ibid., p. 386.

the brain together, this ensemble forms a direct analogy to the enclosed, fluid-filled pregnant womb. To further this analogy, it is interesting to note that an older name for the anterior foramen of the brain's third ventricle is "the vulva" and the quadrigeminal cistern used to be called "the testes".[23] A key to understanding the genesis of the symbolic analogy between the cranium and its contents and the reproductive system might be discovered in the more primitive typology of the Melanesian Trobriand Islanders who have lived in their isolated South Sea habitat for more than 30,000 years. In their explanation of pregnancy, a spirit child comes to rest on the top of a woman's head and when conception occurs, the spirit child flows down through the head in the blood into the womb.[24] If, as the present author believes, these ideas had their genesis in the original African homeland of these people, then this would have been the earliest source of the imagery that connected the brain to the womb. These ideas represent a stage in the progress toward a physiologic conception of pregnancy and though the historic Egyptians were well acquainted with the physiologic nature of conception, they still preserved the earlier ideas as part of their scientific symbolism.

23 Bell, C., *Engravings of the Brain and Nerves,* Birmingham: The Classics of Medicine Library, 1982, pp. 30, 45.

24 Malinowski, B., *The Sexual Life of Savages in Northwestern Melanesia,* London: Routledge & Kegan Paul, 1932, p. 149. The Trobriand Islanders claim that in order for conception to occur, the woman has to "be opened" which is the function of sexual intercourse. This sexual opening is in some way connected to the "opening" (wpt) that occurs on the top of the head which allows the spirit-child to descend to the womb. This relationship is confirmed in a remarkable way by H. E. Sigerist who, on page 113 of his *Primitive and Archaic Medicine,* refers to the discovery in 1895 of a number of *female* skeletons from prehistroic France whose skulls bore "a T-shaped scar beginning on the frontal bone, running all along the sagittal suture, and branching into two parts along the posterior edge of the parietal bones". This would have been a primitive type of "opening" (wpt) of the head as a mode of conception.

Consider the Eye of Horus—a symbol often used in connection with ancient Egyptian culture. In fig. 11, we see a jar used for a medical preparation marked with the *left* Eye of Horus. In fig. 12, the author has compared the left eye of

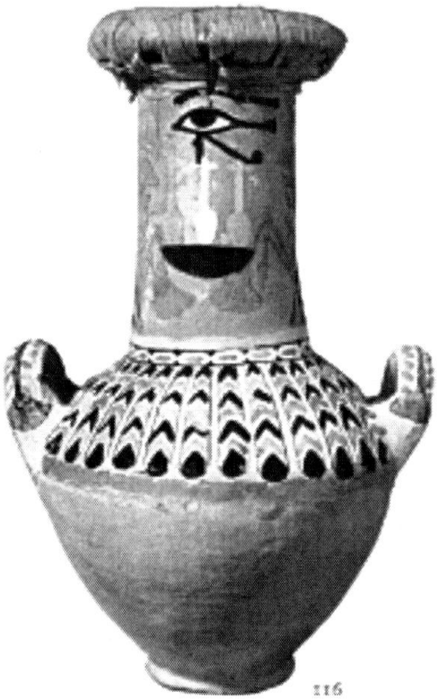

Figure 11
Egyptian Medicine Bottle 1,500 B.C. Emblazoned with the Left Eye of Horus

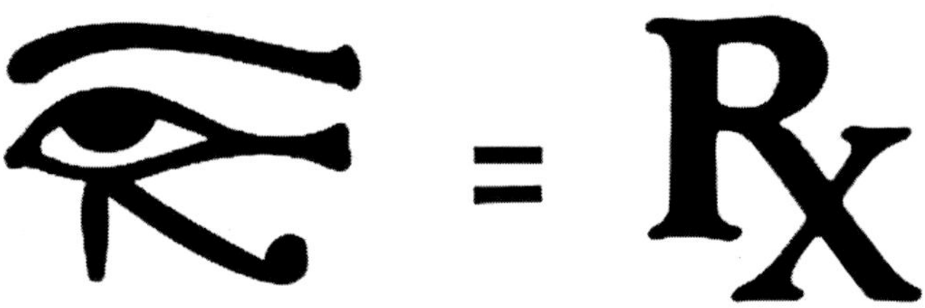

Figure 12
On Left: Left Eye of Horus. On Right: Modern Druggist Symbol

Horus to the current symbol we use to denote a medical prescription or a place where such prescriptions are prepared, i.e., a modern drug store.

ReFaey, et. al. (2019) did an analysis of the brain using the Eye of Horus. They superimposed the Eye of Horus onto the area of the brain below the corpus callosum. Fig. 13. The researchers theorize that each part of the eye of Horus is related to one of the six senses: smell, sight, thought, hearing, taste, and touch. The team goes on to assign each ending of the Eye of Horus to a particular sense using modern knowledge of brain function to validate the location of each sense. Their conclusion is worth noting:

> "Although we recognize the liabilities of overinterpreting a symbolic masterpiece like the Eye of Horus, we propose that the anatomical metaphors in the Eye of Horus are not by coincidence and merit discussion. The ancient Egyptians were leaders in medicine and anatomy. This can be found in documented papyrus, as well as the walls of many temples and tombs. In the creation of Eye of Horus, ancient Egyptians combined their artistic abilities and knowledge of anatomy with their deep belief in mythology. More importantly, we argue that there is a clear influence of their interpretation of human senses on the size and shape of the Eye. This is an amazing feat considering the unavailability of radiographic and computational technology in that era. The significance of our theory of the Eye of Horus is not to be used as an anatomical gold standard but rather to acknowledge and appreciate the genius and foresight of an ancient civilization in decoding the intricate functions of the human central nervous system."[25]

25 ReFaey K, Quinones GC, Clifton W, Tripathi S, and Quinones-Hinojosa A, The Eye of Horus: The Connection Between Art, Medicine, and Mythology in Ancient Egypt. Cureus 2019 May; 11(5):e4731. Doi: 10.7759/cureus.4731 (Reference courtesy of Jewell L. Crawford, M.D.)

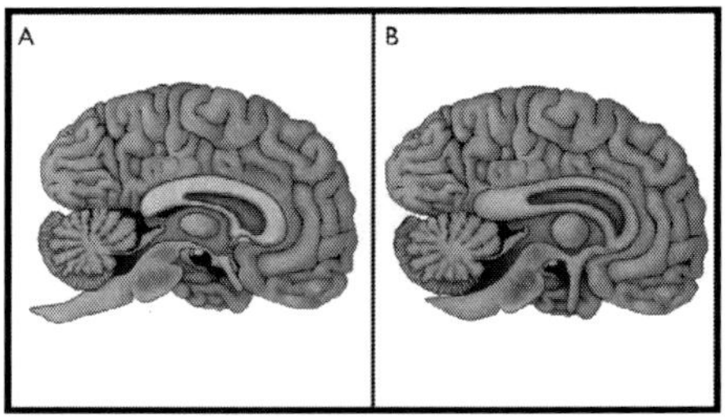

Figure 13a

The human brain in grey color with the corpus callosum, metathalamus, olfactory tract (ReFaey, et al, 2019). *Fig. A shows the actual neuroanatomy Fig. B shows the ancient representation with a slight reposition of the direction of the olfactory tract and a reorientation of the corpus callosum.*

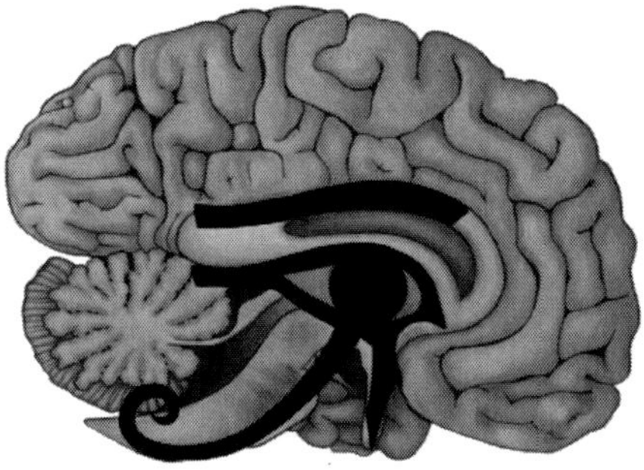

Figure 13b

The Eye of Horus fitted in the mid-sagittal section of the human brain. This figure shows the different parts of the Eye of Horus fitting the anatomical structures that carry special brain function. (ReFaey et al., 2019).

One last point of interest will demonstrate the continuing hold of the ancient symbolism on modern medical science. One of the names of the hippocampus, which is part of the brain's limbic system, is the "Horn of Ammon".[26] The hippocampus is the centre of memory and "Ammon" is the Egyptian Amen,

26 Bell, op. cit., p. 17; also, *Dorland's Medical Dictionary,* Philadelphia: W. B. Saunders, 1974, p. 724.

the ram-headed deity of Thebes. The root of the word "amen" is "men" and this latter, among several meanings, signifies "to be established, to be made firm, to be made permanent", very appropriate meanings for a name denoting the part of the brain that is the memory centre.

A few selected cases of the 48 recorded in the Edwin Smith Papyrus can now be considered to illustrate the scope of Egyptian medical knowledge.[27] It will be noted, as we proceed through this discussion, that this ancient physician adopts a clinical method almost identical to our own involving an examination, a diagnosis, a prognosis, and a treatment (if indicated); all of this some 35 centuries before Hippocrates.

The first case under consideration is Case 6. The reader will note that the case description is written in a characteristically concise, though figurative, style which is nonetheless clinical in tone. It is in this case that are first met the terms for "meninges" and "cerebrospinal fluid" as well as a description of the external appearance of the brain. The glosses are the explanatory notes, appended by the 18th dynasty editor, necessary to properly understand the archaic language.

Case Six: A Gaping Wound In The Head With Compound Comminuted Fracture Of The Skull And Rupture Of The Meningeal Membranes

Examination: If thou examinest a man having a gaping wound in his head, penetrating to the bone, smashing his skull, and rending open the brain of his skull, thou shouldst palpate his wound. Shouldst thou find that smash which is in his skull like

27 All of the following cases cited are taken from the Classics of Medicine Library edition of Breasted's translation. See Note 12.

those corrugations which form in molten copper, and something therein throbbing and fluttering under thy fingers, like the weak place of an infant's crown before it becomes whole—when it has happened there is no throbbing and fluttering under thy fingers until the brain of his skull is rent open—and he discharges blood from both his nostrils, and he suffers with stiffness in his neck.

Diagnosis: Thou shouldst say concerning him: "An ailment not to be treated".

Treatment: Thou shouldst anoint that wound with grease. Thou shalt not bind it; thou shalt not apply two strips upon it; until thou knowest he has reached a decisive point.

Gloss A: As for—"Smashing his skull, and rending open the brain of his skull", it means the smash is large, opening to the interior of his skull, to the membrane enveloping his brain, so that it breaks open his fluid into the interior of his head.

Gloss B: As for—"Those corrugations which form on molten copper", it means copper which the coppersmith pours off before it is forced into the mold, because of something foreign upon it like wrinkles. It is said: "It is like ripples of pus".

Gloss A shows us conclusively that the author is denoting the meninges when he speaks of the "membrane ('netnet') enveloping his brain". Moreover, he establishes their relation to the cerebrospinal fluid when he writes, "it breaks open the fluid into the interior of his head", meaning that the rupture of the meninges caused by the blow causes the fluid within it to flow into the cranial cavity. Gloss B gives us an unmistakable description of the convolutions of the brain which in fact do resemble " corrugations which form on molten copper". The Examination, describing the haemorrhage through the nostrils with stiffness of the neck, is clinically on target. Any skull fracture due to penetrating trauma can very readily result in bleeding through the nose. The stiffness of the neck can be the result of two possible complications: 1) meningeal inflammation (meningitis) due to the invasion of the cerebrospinal structures by external micro-organisms or 2) bleeding into the nuchal (posterior neck) segment of the spinal cord. As the surgeon notes here when he concludes that this is "An ailment not to be treated", these are both prognostically grave signs.

The next case, Case 8, presents a fascinating discussion of a rather rare neurosurgical condition, the"contre-coup" cranial injury. To understand this properly it must be pointed out that the motor and sensory fibers that control most voluntary movement and sensation actually arise on the side of the brain opposite to the side they control. This means that the movement and feeling on the left side of the body is controlled by the right side of the brain and that of the right side of the body by the left side of the brain. The term "contre-coup" means that the force of a blow on one side of the skull is transmitted and causes injury to the opposite side of the brain. The effects of this injury will be felt on the side of the skull to which the blow was delivered rather than, as might be expected, the opposite side. We might note here, by the way, that this description of a contre-coup injury makes it almost certain that we are dealing here with the work of a battlefield surgeon since this is precisely the kind of injury that would be caused by a club striking the side of the head.

Case Eight: Compound Comminuted Fracture Of The Skull Displaying No Visible External Injury.

Examination: If thou examinest a man having a smash of his skull, under the skin of his head, while there is nothing at all upon it, thou shouldst palpate his wound. Shouldst thou find that there is a swelling protruding on the outside of that smash which is in his skull, while his eye is askew because of it, on the side of him having that injury which is in his skull; and he walks shuffling with his sole, on the side of him having that injury which is in his skull...

Diagnosis: Thou shouldst account him one who something entering from outside has smitten, as one who does not release the head of his shoulder fork, and one who does not fall with his nails in the middle of his palm; while he discharges blood from both his nostrils and from both his ears, and he suffers with stiffness in his neck. An ailment not to be treated.

Treatment: His treatment is sitting, until he gains colour, and until thou knowest he has reached the decisive point.

Second Examination: Now as soon as thou findest that smash which is in his skull like those corrugations which form on molten copper, and something therein throbbing and fluttering under thy fingers like the weak place of an infant's crown before it knits together—when it has happened there is no throbbing and fluttering under thy fingers, until the brain of his skull is rent open—and he discharges blood from both his nostrils and both his ears, and he suffers with stiffness in his neck...

Second Diagnosis: Thou shouldst say concerning him: "An ailment not to be treated."

Gloss A: As for—"A smash in his skull under the skin of his head, there being no wound at all upon it," it means a smash of the shell of his skull, the flesh of his head being uninjured.

Gloss B: As for—"He walks with shuffling with his sole," he (the surgeon) is speaking about his walking with his sole dragging, so that it is not easy for him to walk when the sole is feeble and turned over, while the tips of his toes are contracted to the ball of his sole, and the toes walking fumbling the ground. The surgeon says: "He shuffles," concerning it.

Gloss C: As for—"One whom something entering from outside has smitten", on the side of him having this injury, it means one whom something entering from outside presses, on the side of him having this injury.

The modern clinician can only read these case presentations with amazement and admiration. The ability to relate a specific trauma to a complex set of neurological signs and symptoms as we see here is the mark of a physician whose clinical acumen has been developed to the highest degree. The physician was well aware that an illness had a natural history which underwent exacerbations and remissions before the final outcome became conclusive. This is indicated in this case by virtue of the second examination. In fact in Case 7, the surgeon records his findings and opinions which are derived from yet a third examination. In the Second Examination of this case we seem to have the only known Egyptian reference to the procedure of trephination when the patient's skull is said to be "rent open". Trephination, practiced extensively throughout Africa since prehistoric times, is a method in which an instrument is used to bore through the skull to remove bony fragments from a fracture or to relieve cranial pressure. Many have doubted that the Egyptians actually used this technique but Paul Ghalioungui has reproduced photos of two trephined skulls from an Egyptian gravesite.[28] If we are correct in assuming, after Breasted,[29] that it is trephining being referred to in this case, then it is additional proof that this technique was a part of the therapeutic armamentarium of ancient Egyptian physicians.

Gloss B gives a lucid and painstaking description of the shuffling gait with contractures of the toes, indicative of a hemi-paresis or severe motor weakness, caused by this contrecoup injury. Then, as now, the mainstay of care was supportive treatment.

Finally it must be pointed out that when the surgeon says, "his eye is askew", as a result of this injury he seems to be referring to damage to the oculomotor nerve, one of three controlling eye movements.[30] Again, the remarkable thing to note is the way in which the surgeon correctly relates a specific event (head trauma) to a neurological outcome.

Case 20 is one of four in which the surgeon demonstrates his knowledge of the relationship between injuries to the temporal portion of the brain and the faculty of speaking. In the anterior

28 See Ghalioungui, op. cit., plates 15 a and b, after p. 122.

29 Breasted, op. cit., pp. 56, 208.

30 The three cranial nerves controlling eye movements are the oculomotor (III), the trochlear (IV), and the abducens (VI). According to my neurologist informant, Dr. Patrick Griffith, the oculomotor and the trochlear are the most likely to be affected by blunt trauma to the temporal region, causing the eye to skew.

portion of the temporal region of the brain lies Broca's area which is the motor centre of speech. An injury or lesion here affects the patient's ability to properly articulate words, though he will understand what is being said. Behind Broca's area is Wernicke's area which is the receptive centre of speech; a lesion here affects the patient's ability to understand the spoken word though the purely mechanical ability to form words remains untouched. Persons affected in Wernicke's area will speak coherently but in meaningless, non-sensical phrases. A speech problem affecting Broca's area is known as "expressive aphasia" and that in Wernicke's area as "receptive aphasia". Not uncommonly, a temporal lesion will affect both areas causing a "mixed" or "total" aphasia.

Case Twenty: A Wound In The Temple Perforating The Bone

Examination: If thou examinest a man having a wound in his temple, penetrating to the bone, and perforating his temporal bone, while his two eyes are bloodshot, he discharges blood from both his nostrils, and a little drops; if thou puttest thy finger on the mouth of that wound he shudders exceedingly; if thou ask of him concerning his malady and he speaketh not to thee; while copious tears fall from both his eyes, so that he thrusts his hand often to his face that he may wipe both his eyes with the back of his hand as a child does, and does not know that he does so...

Diagnosis: Thou shouldst say concerning him: "One having a wound in his temple, penetrating to the bone, and perforating his temporal bone; while he discharges blood from both his nostrils, he suffers with stiffness in his neck, and he is speechless. An ailment not to be treated".

The patient is unable to verbally respond to the surgeon's interrogation which shows that the surgeon recognizes this as an expressive aphasia caused by an injury to the temporal portion of the brain. The tearing of the eyes is a very interesting sign. Trauma to the temple can result in a facial nerve injury causing increased tearing in the eye on the involved side. But our ancient surgeon is very explicit about the presence of *bilateral* tearing. Individuals suffering from an expressive aphasia will often become so frustrated at their inability to speak properly that they will burst into tears.[31] As for the repetitious movements of the hand to the eyes, Schwaller de Lubicz considers this an example of an "apraxia", a neurological sign characterized by meaningless, unconscious movements.[32]

Case 22 is very similar to Case 20 and seems to describe a total aphasia. In the Examination, the Surgeon says concerning the patient, "If thou callest to him and he is speechless and cannot speak...", which may indicate an absolute incapacity for speech such as would be true of total aphasia. However, Schwaller de Lubicz gives another possible interpretation of this locution. Looking at Gloss C, it states: "As for—'He is speechless', it means that he is silent in sadness, without speaking, like one suffering with feebleness (prostration?) because of something that has entered from outside". The combination of speechlessness and "silent in sadness" may refer to a kind of mental obtundation that would justify us in thinking, as Schwaller de Lubicz believes, that this patient is in a coma.[33] Whatever the case, it is difficult not

31 The author would like to express his gratitude to Dr. Patrick Griffith for his comments on this material.

32 Schwaller de Lubicz, op. cit., p. 622.

33 I id., pp. 623–24.

to believe that the ancient Egyptian physicians, on the basis of the evidence presented here, identified and possibly even mapped the location and function of certain important cortical centres of the brain, a feat not to be achieved again until the 19th century.

Case 31 is one of a group (Cases 29–33) which demonstrates further the uncommon level of clinical expertise achieved by this ancient surgeon. He describes in accurate detail the catastrophic clinical consequences of a certain type of spinal cord injury.

Case Thirty-One: Dislocation Of A Cervical Vertebra

Examination: If thou examinest a man having a dislocation in a vertebra of his neck, shouldst thou find him unconscious of his two arms and his two legs on account of it, while his phallus is erected on account of it, and urine drops from his member without knowing it; his flesh has received wind; his two eyes are blood-shot; it is a dislocation of a vertebra of his neck extending to his backbone which causes him to be unconscious of his two arms and his two legs. If, however, the middle vertebra of his neck is dislocated, it is an "emissio seminis" which befalls his phallus.

Diagnosis: Thou shouldst say concerning him: "One having a dislocation in a vertebra of his neck, while he is unconscious of his two legs and his two arms, and his urine dribbles. An ailment not to be treated."

Gloss A: As for—"A dislocation in a vertebra of his neck", he is speaking of a separation of one vertebra of his neck from another, the flesh which is over it being uninjured; as one says, "It is wnkh", concerning things which had been joined together, when one has been severed from another.

Gloss B: As for—"It is an 'emissio seminis' which befalls his phallus", it means that his phallus is erected and has a discharge from the end of his phallus. It is said: "It remains stationary" (mn saw), when it cannot sink downward and it cannot lift upward.

Gloss C: As for—"While his urine dribbles", it means that urine drops from his phallus and cannot hold back for him.

The language is so simple and concise that it may not be easy to appreciate the mine of clinical information contained in this case description. First there is a completely accurate description of quadriplegia ("unconscious of his two arms and his two legs") resulting from a compression injury to the cervical spinal cord due to a spinal dislocation. Though not specified, it is thought that this compression occurs below the 4th cervical vertebra because breathing remains intact.[34] The descriptions of the genitourinary complications are very striking for our surgeon delineates priapism, spermatorrhea, and bladder incontinence as complications of this condition. Can it not be assumed that he knew that the physiological sexual response and the urinary functions are mediated through the spinal cord?[35] Such things did not become known to modern medicine until the last century. One

34 Ibid., p. 588.

35 One of the errors for which Greek medicine is repeatedly called to task is the idea that male sperm is formed in the spinal cord. This idea was very likely due to a misinterpretation of the Egyptians' clinical description of "emissio seminis" that results from a spinal cord injury.

other phrase from this Case begs explanation and that is the reference in the Examination to the fact that "his flesh has received wind". If a quadriplegic patient experiences a prolonged survival, his body becomes thick and soft. Schwaller de Lubicz is of the opinion that this phrase "his flesh has received wind" refers to the "insufflation" effect that occurs in the quadriplegic body.[36]

Cases 29–33 all represent additional case descriptions of vertebral dislocations and sub-luxations and their clinical consequences. At present, some of these conditions are almost impossible to detect or describe fully without X-ray studies. The question then arises is how did our ancient surgeon, living and practicing 6,000 years ago, manage to diagnose and describe these problems *without* benefit of X-rays?

A tour through the Edwin Smith Papyrus puts us in the rather incongruous position of having to assert that as history dawns in the Nile Valley at the end of the 5th millenium B.C., medicine is already at a very advanced state and that in fact, it underwent a decline in later ages which was not reversed until the scientific breakthroughs of the 18th and 19th centuries. It is the conceit of modern historiography that human culture has evolved in linear fashion from the simple to the complex, from the primitive to the advanced, from the lower to the higher, reaching its pinnacle in the post-Renaissance civilization of Western Europe. A more clear-sighted perception of history would show us that this idea flies in the face of the true facts. The progression of human civilization might be more accurately described as a sinusoidal wave, in which the ebb and flow of civilized progress is represented by peaks and valleys. From every pinnacle there is a

36 Schwaller de Lubicz, op. cit., p. 589.

regression and every succeeding civilization is faced with having to re-discover old truths. The Greek "miracle" is but the detritus of ancient Egyptian thought and many of the "marvels" of the modern age are the fruit of recovering older ideas. But this recovery is only partial. Schwaller de Lubicz calls modern science "a science without illumination" because it has consciously forfeited the dynamic interplay between science and symbol which made Egyptian wisdom proverbial throughout the ancient world.

CHAPTER FOUR

African Traditional Healing—Superstition, Savagery, or Science?

One has little or no idea of the power that resides in Africa; even most Africans in Africa seem oblivious to it. African traditional healing methods are probably among some of the least understood of the world's healing practices. Labeled primitive, demonic, and dangerous, these traditions have not often been included in the recent re-examination and resurgence of traditional healing systems from Chinese, Hindu, and Native American cultures. The word, "Voodoo," for example, still has very negative, lurid connotations because it is seen primarily as a practice of dark arts. The current popular fascination with zombies is a direct outgrowth, since the fear inspired by voodoo practitioners was their reputed ability to turn normal persons into mindless, soulless zombies. And this morbid fascination with these bizarre doings goes hand-in-hand with what people believe about "black magic" or witchcraft. Is there such a thing?

It must be stated, however, that traditional African belief systems have a dual nature; they CAN be directed into a force for harm. Says author, J. Olumide Lucas, "Ancient magic was the very foundation of religion."[1]

1 Lucas, J.Olumide, *The Religion of the Yourubas*, J. Olumide Lucas/Lucas Estate, 1966, p. 267

> 'Positive' magic assumes the forms of sorcery, exercise of mysterious powers *for good* ***or*** *ill* (author's emphasis), use of charms and practice of occultism for therapeutic ***or*** *other purposes* (author's emphasis), and performances based on a claim to possession of esoteric and mysterious knowledge.[2]

The spiritual leaders in Africa were individuals who were highly trained, very often from childhood. We could describe these men and women as "adepts," or magicians because they learned how to manipulate energy. The priests/magicians of Egypt did not share the sacred knowledge except with other priests and initiates because of its power. These magician priests were bound under the highest moral authority in the practice of their work. At some point in history, some sub-set of these priests or magicians began to use the ancient sacred practices and secrets for personal gain and control--even for evil and inimical purposes. Now we have dark magic or witchcraft. And this ability—for good and for ill—can be found everywhere in the world. The fundamental point is that power—like money—corrupts. Indeed, even modern science and medical practices can be used in negative ways. Atomic energy, for example, can be used for bombs, or to power electricity. This is the reason why for hundreds of years, physicians and healers have taken solemn oaths to "do no harm" before they can begin to practice.

The practices crossed the Atlantic as Africans were enslaved. In her book, *Working Cures*, Sharla Fett describes numerous examples of "conjuring" or the use of traditional African systems by the enslaved to intentionally do harm to others.[3] Full ceremo-

2 Ibid., p.268

3 Fett, S.M., *Working Cures, Healing health, and power on southern slave plantations,* Chapel Hill, University of North Carolina Press, 2002, pp. 84–108.

nies and drumming were banned by slaveholders out of fear of this power. Individual enslaved healers (who were often women) learned how to use other aspects of their African traditions to heal including prayer, dedicated bedside nursing (which we now call "therapeutic presence"), amulets for healing or protection, and an extensive knowledge of plant pharmacology. These healers quietly preserved and continued African healing practices in ways more 'acceptable' to their owners.[4]

Let us now examine the components of African traditional belief systems when they are used for their highest good—healing for the individual and the community. These systems integrate all of the forces that impact human life into a harmonious balance. Healing interventions operate on multiple levels—biophysical, psychic, energetic, spiritual, and cosmic—interacting seamlessly within a multi-dimentional model of the human self. In Africa, the philosophy of "I am because we are" highlights the indispensable role of a healthy community, both spiritually and materially, in ensuring the health of the individual. In other words, the health of the individual is dependent on the health and well-being of the community at large. This communal aspect of health challenges the more individualistic approach often seen in Western medicine and reiterates the importance of harmony and balance across all planes of existence. By examining the multi-dimensional African spiritual personality alongside the African family model, we can appreciate that the distinction between spirit and matter in Western scientific thought is artificial. There is a seamless continuum between these states through a "ladder of energy," making it impossible to live properly with-

4 Ibid., pp.111–141, p. 196

out engaging in both realms. Illness can be viewed as a dialogue between Spirit and man. *Healing* restores the balance of all forces impacting human life—as opposed to *curing*, which addresses mostly physical distress to restore a sense of well-being. In Africa, healing rites and initiatory rites are often the same, as healing transforms and initiates the individual.

In most traditional African systems, healing requires the intervention of one or more spirits or "higher" powers. The system of the Vodũ is a traditional belief system of the Fon and Ewe peoples of Benin and Togo. The Vodũ are the spiritual Powers, of which there are 41 major ones. Their direct counterparts elsewhere in Africa are the *neters* of ancient Egypt, the *rabs* of the Senegalese Lebu, the abosom of the Akan of Ghana, the *nommo* of the Dogon of Mali, and the *orishas* of the Nigerian Yoruba. The destinies of the Universe and of humanity are directed by these Powers.

An African model of the self, as described by Dr. Erick Gbodossou of Benin, includes spiritual/cosmic, energetic, moral/religious, psychic/emotional, and biophysical dimensions.[5] For an individual to be in a state of total health, all these dimensions must be in harmony and balance. Imbalance in any one dimension indicates incomplete health. In this schema, the biophysical dimension, which is the primary focus of modern Western medicine, is the *smallest* and *least significant*. Thus, physical well-being,

5 Gbodossou, Erick V.A. *The African Concept from God to Man: An Introduction to African Spiritualism*, 2004, Prometra International, Dakar, Senegal, p. 13

Erick Gbodossou is a practicing physician born and raised in Benin—the epicenter of the old empire of Dahomey. He lives and works just outside of Dakar, Senegal. Under the tutelage of his grandfather he was deeply instructed in the world system of the Vodũ. He is, therefore, knowledgeable about modern AND traditional medicine. He is the founder and President of PROMETRA International—Promotion des Médecines Traditionelles

while essential, is not sufficient for overall health. The true task for humans is to strive for unity and integration of all human dimensions, achieving both health and freedom.

An African Model of the Self

Erick Gbodossou

Spiritual Cosmic

Energetic

Moral Religious

Pyschic Emotional

Biophysical

The Self is the Nexus through which the visible and invisible units of the family conjoin in a Crossing. That is the reason why crossing symbols—especially the crossroads—are so important in African psycho-spiritual life. The point of intersection at the crossroads is the place where the physical meets the spiritual. Future descendants are not referred to as "unborn," but as the "yet-to-be-born," existing on a vertical continuum with ancestors. The yet-to-be-born and the ancestors are, in effect, the same. This reciprocal web of relations connects the living with the living; the living with the invisible relations, i.e., the ancestors and the yet-to-be-born; and finally connects the two invisible relations—those of the past, and those of the future.[6] Related to this web of relations is the profoundly African concept that "the dead are not dead." Among

6 Ibid, pp.21–22.)

the Dogon, maintaining these connections is so important that neglecting ancestral duties can lead to spiritual and social upheaval.

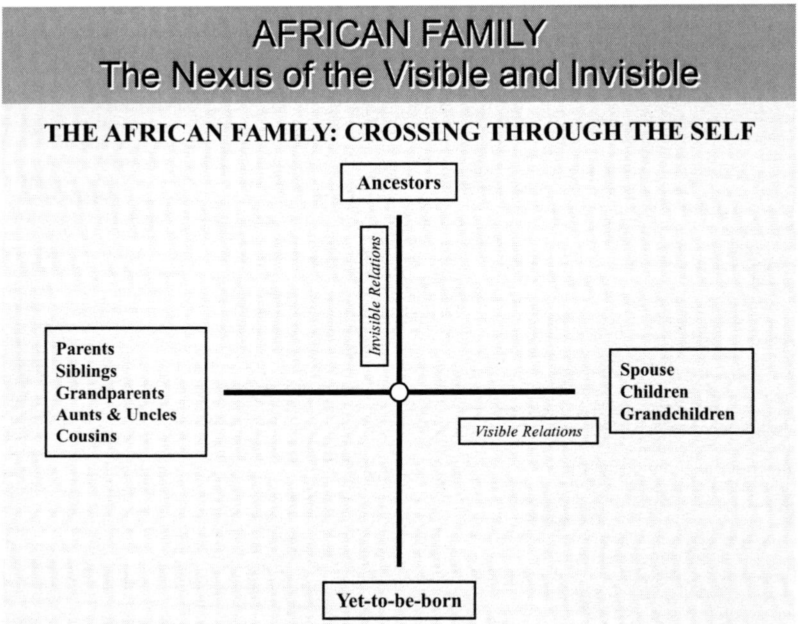

In African spiritual traditions, the universe is believed to have originated as a thought in the Mind of the Creator, brought into existence through the power of the Word. This profound essence of African traditional medicine can be encapsulated in the powerful concept: "In the beginning was the Word." This conceptualization holds that words are not merely sounds or symbols, but active, potent forces capable of shaping reality. Historically, African societies have recognized the inherent power of words, exercising great caution in their use, mindful that even casual utterances could manifest real-world consequences. The sacredness attributed to the spoken word is particularly evident in the domain of healing, where prayers and incantations form the cornerstone of therapeutic practices. Often a prayer offered by a spiritually powerful individual is, by itself, sufficient to effect a successful healing outcome. This reverence for the spoken word aligns with the broader African medicinal philosophy, which is holistic and integrative; transcending the mere biophysical to include psychic, energetic, spiritual, and cosmic dimensions.

The role of the healer in African societies often blurs the lines between a physician and a priest, reflecting a historical unity that was prevalent across many cultures worldwide. This unity acknowledges that *healing the body* cannot be divorced from *healing the spirit.* 350 years ago, Reneé Descartes, a French philosopher and mathematician introduced the concept of 'doubt' into scientific thinking, making science more empirical and experiment-driven. This shift led to a focus on observation and scientific trials in medicine, often excluding faith and prayer. The Flexner Report (1910) further cemented this shift in America by advocating a strong basic sciences curriculum as the foundation for medical training, relegating religion and spirituality to irrelevance in medical practice.[7] Traditional African healing integrates spiritual and medicinal practices seamlessly in ceremonies and individual encounters.

The resurgence of interest in traditional practices, reflects a cyclic return to these holistic approaches. This movement, gaining momentum in the United States since the early 1990s, has seen a significant embrace of practices like homeopathy, chiropractic, and herbal remedies, which are now being integrated into mainstream medical curricula as complementary therapies.

7 Flexner, Abraham, *Medical Education in the United States and Canada: A Report To the Carnegie Foundation For the Advancement of Teaching.* New York, NY, USA: The Carnegie Foundation for the Advancement of Teaching; 1910. [PMC free article] [PubMed] [Google Scholar]

- Homeopathy is a system that relies on infinitesimal doses of remedies that in normal concentrations would produce the symptoms of the disease being treated. The active ingredient of homeopathic remedies often is present in such small concentrations that it is undetectable by laboratory analysis.
- Phytomedicine (plant medicine) has assumed ever greater importance because somewhere between 25 and 30% of the drugs used in our modern pharmacopeia are derived from the plant kingdom. These include digitalis, cocaine, ipecac, aspirin, curare, atropine, ephedrine, tetracycline, penicillin, colchicine, physostigmine, reserpine, and morphine, to name just a handful of modern drugs.
- The effect of prayer and religious belief on health outcomes is being re-evaluated. Studies are showing that patients actively engaged in prayer regularly have much better recovery times and outcomes than those who aren't.[8]
- Acupuncture's efficacy has been well proven; endorphins released by nerve stimulation, are known to be the biochemical mediators accounting for the effects of acupuncture, especially in anesthesia.

Medical schools have established holistic/complementary medicine programs. The term, 'alternative medicine ' is being replaced with the phrase, 'integrative medicine.' Modern medicine has begun to recognize the need to include ancient therapies to bring about a more complete—or holistic—healing for patients.

This renaissance of ancient healing wisdom will soon find its way into the re-evaluation of African spiritual and medic-

8 Guarneri, M, *The Heart Speaks A cardiologist reveals the secret language of healing,* 2006, Touchstone, New York, pp. 118–122.

inal practices, which offer rich models of human health that are multi-dimensional. These models incorporate a spectrum of human experience from the spiritual and cosmic to the biophysical, advocating for a balanced existence that synchronizes all aspects of being. It becomes clear that the ancient African insight into the power of the word, the importance of community, and the interconnectedness of all aspects of life, provides not only a window into the past but a promising direction for the future of holistic health care. It is for this reason that the author has chosen to explore the philosophical underpinnings of African medicine but also illustrate its practical applications, showing how ancient traditions can inform and enrich modern therapeutic practices.

Let us now examine two ethnic groups in Senegal who continue to practice their traditional belief systems for healing, the Serer and the Lebu peoples of Senegal.

The Serer are one of Senegal's five major ethnic groups, living in the Fatick region of west-central Senegal. The are closely allied ethnically and culturally to the Lebu. Their oral history suggests that they arrived in Senegal many centuries ago from lands bordering the Nile. Even today, the Serer are not completely Islamized, and have maintained their ancient, traditional spiritual and healing system more-or-less intact. They acknowledge a Supreme Creator named *Roog Sen*, and a multitude of Powers that emanate from Him. The Powers are called *pangool,* a word also meaning 'serpents.' *Roog Sen* governs the workings and destiny of the universe through the *pangool*; and *Roog Sen* is often represented in Serer iconography by the 5-pointed star.

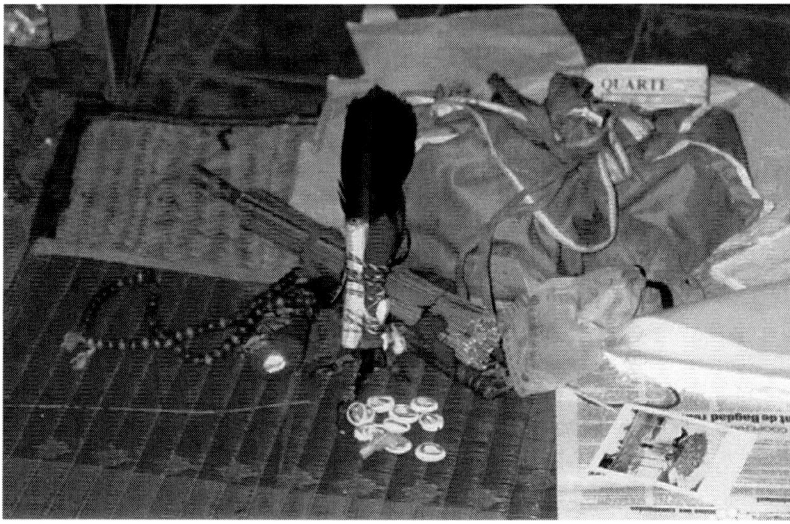

Figure 1
Saltigue's herbs and power objects.
Photo courtesy of Virginia Davis Floyd, M.D.

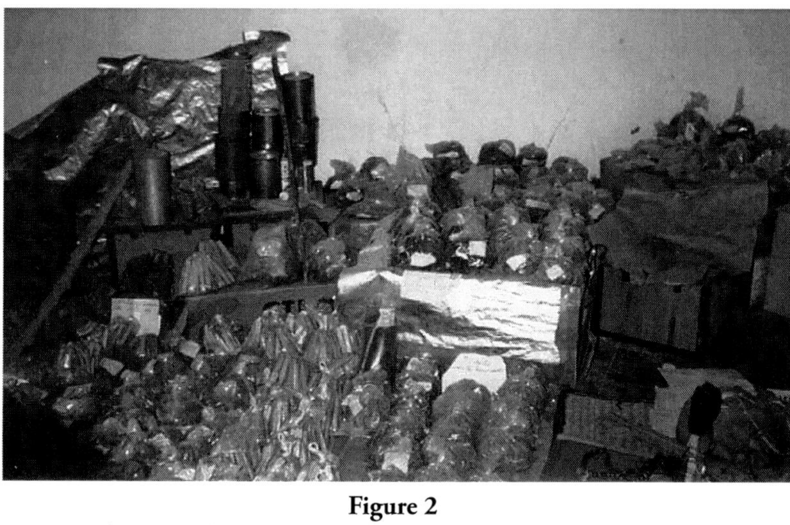

Figure 2
Saltigue Herbs. Photo courtesy of Virginia Davis Floyd, M.D.

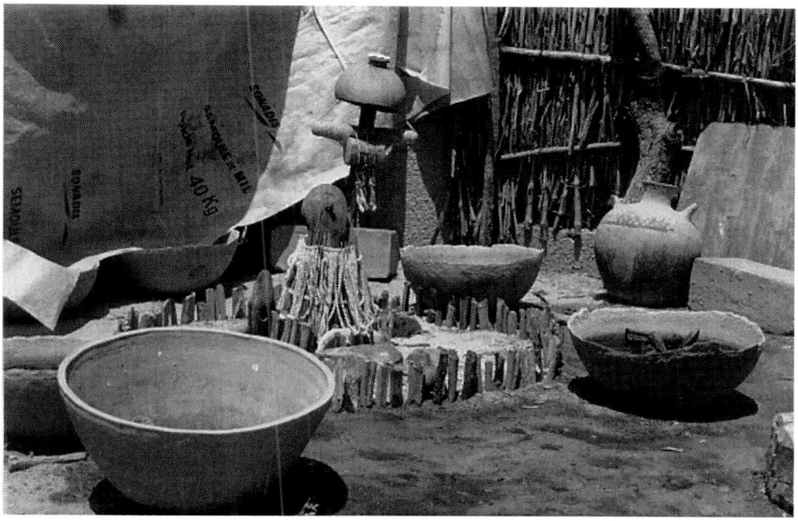

Figure 3
Saltigue's ritual paraphenalia.
Photo courtesy of Virginia Davis Floyd, M.D.

Like all traditional African societies, the Serer accomplish their healing work through the ancestors and the spirits, while extensively utilizing plants and herbs. Their healers are also their priests, and must assume responsibility for the well-being of the whole community. Every June, the priest-healers, called *saltigues,* conduct a ceremony called a *khoye*. At this event, which lasts 2 to 3 days, the *saltigues* foretell the future for the community, the country, and even the wider world. If the future holds unhappy tidings for the community, rites and sacrifices are then conducted to forestall them. The Serer, under the impetus of Erick Gbodossou, M.D., organized the Malango Traditional Healers' Association with its own healing center in Fatick. Since it opened in 1989, thousands of clients have come through Malango Healing Center.

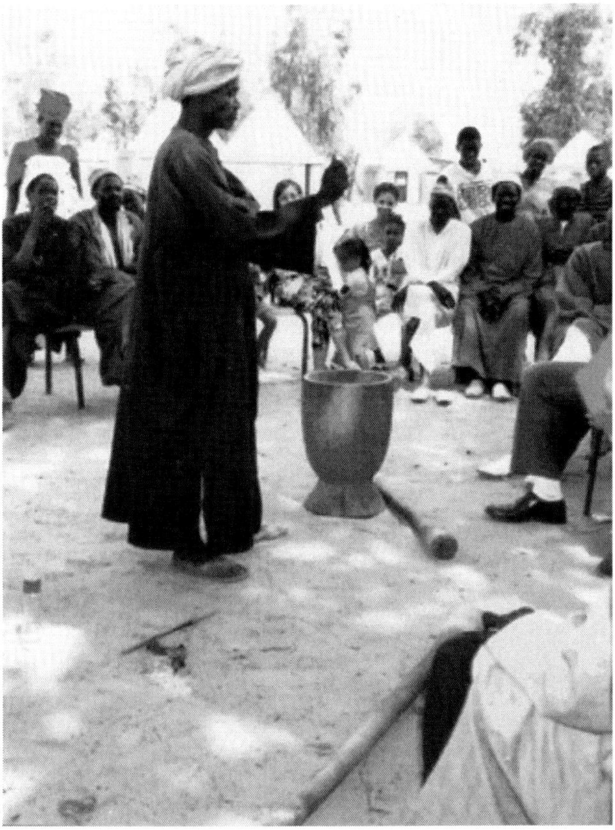

Figure 4
***Saltigue at Malango.* Photo courtesy of Virginia Davis Floyd, M.D.**

The Lebu are a major Senegalese ethnic group with cultural linkages to the Serer. They live on Senegal's Atlantic coast. Their oral history says that they used to live in what is now Libya; and their name, Lebu, was the ancient Egyptian name for Libya. More strongly and pervasively Islamic than the Serer, the Lebu have nevertheless preserved their ancient pre-Islamic spiritual healing system, *Ndepp. Ndepp* is controlled by practitioners called *Ndeppkats,* 90% of whom are women. The Lebu have a

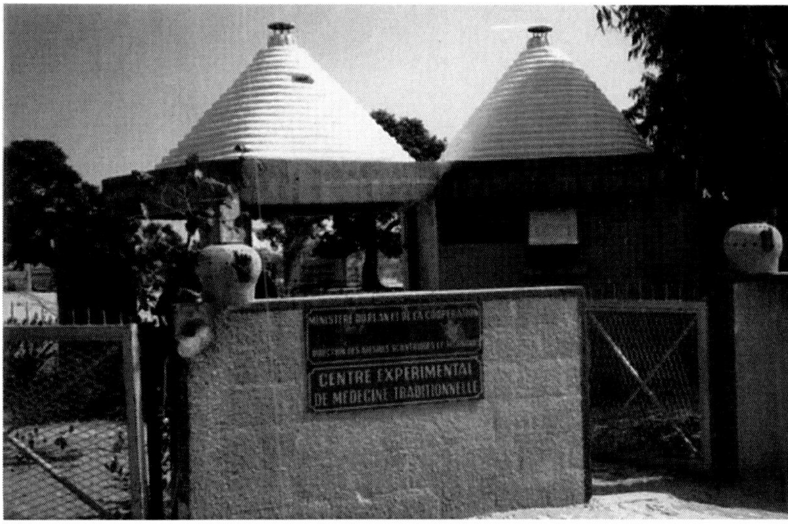

Figure 5
Experimental Center for Traditional Medicine at Malango (Fatick, Senegal).
Photo courtesy of Virginia Davis Floyd, M.D.

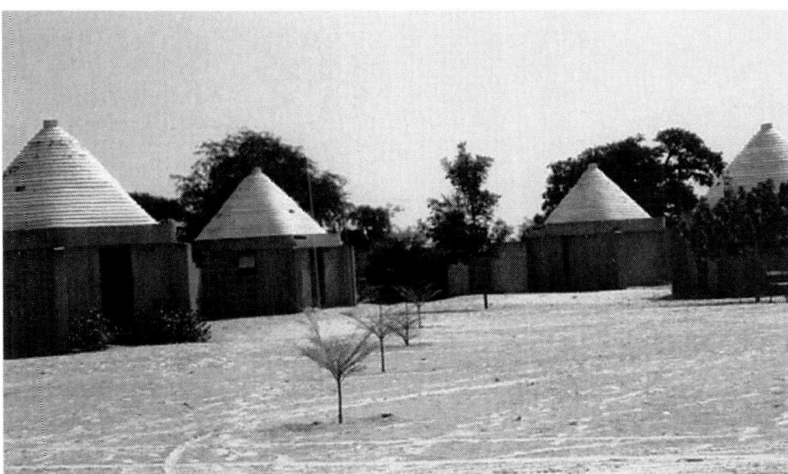

Figure 6
Healing dispensaries at Malango.
Photo courtesy of Virginia Davis Floyd, M.D.

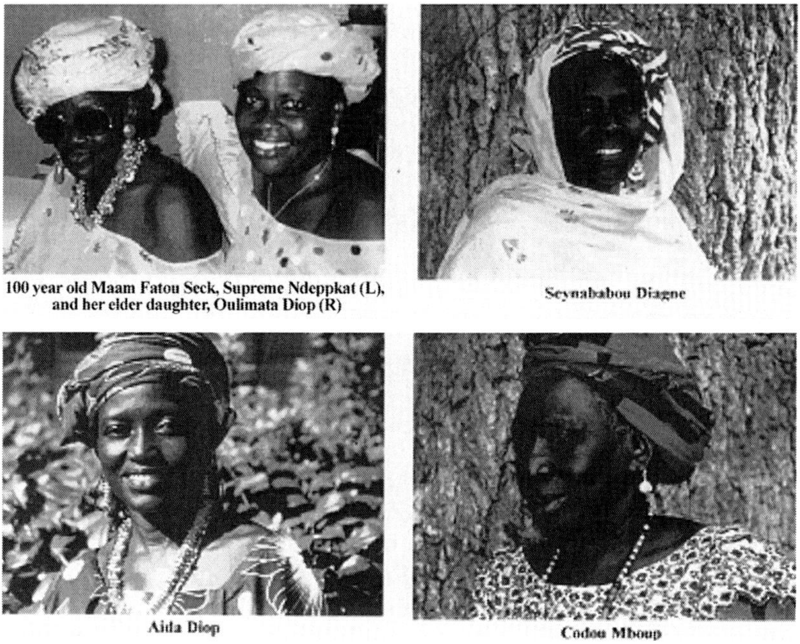

100 year old Maam Fatou Seck, Supreme Ndeppkat (L), and her elder daughter, Oulimata Diop (R)

Seynabalbou Diagne

Aida Diop

Codou Mboup

Figure 7
Ndeppkats. **Photos by Lenny Foster.**

spiritual pantheon which they call *rabs*. The *rabs* are the exact equivalent of the Serer *pangool*. They are the cosmo-spiritual and ancestral beings of *ndepp*. The number of *rabs* is vast, but there are seven major ones:

- *Maam Coumba Lamba,* the Leader of ALL the *rabs,* ruler of the ocean, veritably the Great Mother of the Waters.
- *Matuley Faye*, the *rab* of Muslims, whose element is the earth
- *Ndiare*, the daughter of Coumba Lamba, and the *rab* of pools, lagoons, and rivers
- *Nak Dawur Mbaye*, whose symbol is the serpent, and who rules over Dakar, the capital city of Senegal.

- *Maam Nguessou,* the *rab* of griots and drummers.
- *Mbassi,* the *rab* of trees
- *Maam Massamba Ndoye*, the messenger *rab* and lover of spiritous beverages

The Lebu insist that the *rabs* are not worshipped. Only Allah can be worshipped, but the *rabs* are venerated. Since they do Allah's will, they are asked to intervene and help in alleviating health issues and sorting out the difficulties of everyday life. The *rabs* are especially effective in healing disorders of the mind and spirit. Most such disorders are attributed to wrongdoing, or inappropriate behavior, either social or religious. The *Ndeppkats* show that psychic and physical disturbances flow from spiritual etiologies, which determine the behavior and actions of human beings. All African healing systems employ divination methods to ascertain the cause or causes of psycho-spiritual derangements, and *Ndepp* is no exception. *Ndeppkats* throw cowrie shells on a straw mat, most commonly. They receive information through the cowries, such as whether the person to be healed requires a sacrifice; and if so, what kind. Similarly, in Swaziland, the Sangomas (healers) throw a variety of objects including shells, bones, dominoes, dice, coins, and stones onto a mat. They divine by reading the pattern of these objects after they are thrown and relate the patterns to the ill person. The Sangoma may suggest treatments such as a bath, or a sacrifice.

Ndepp healing ceremonies involve drumming, dancing, and singing to communicate with and summon the *rabs.* Each *rab* has specific rhythms and songs, and master drummers spend years perfecting them. The drum rhythms will summon the *rabs* into the community of devotees. In tandem with the drumming

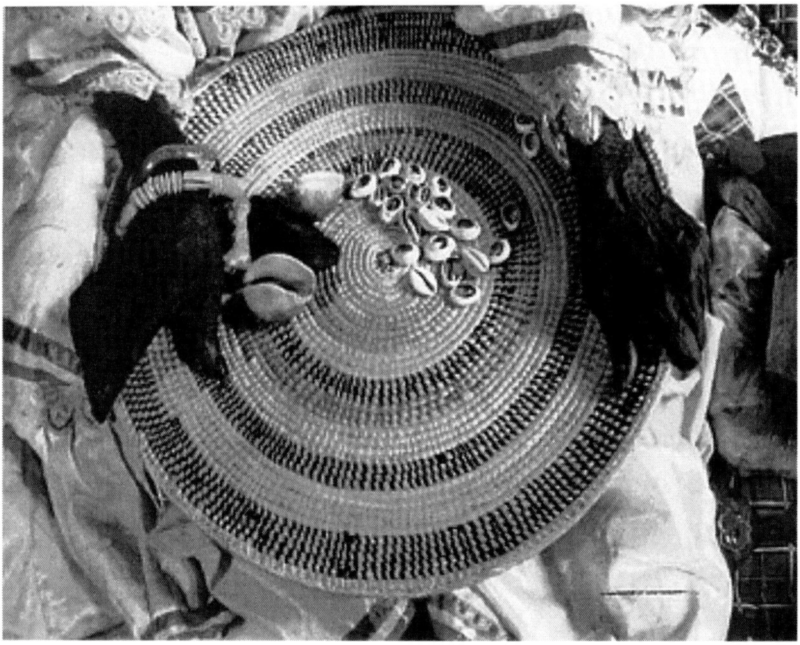

Figure 8
Ndepp cowrie shell divination. **Photo by Lenny Foster.**

comes the dance. The more vigorous and heartfelt the dancing, the more pleasing it is to the *rab.* Dancing, therefore, is an act of worship, a bodily prayer, so to speak. The devotees sing as they dance. The drum rhythms, dances, and songs all work in synergy and harmony to summon the *rabs.* The lead *Ndeppkat* offers prayers on behalf of individuals, families, or the entire community. It is believed that the *rabs* convey the patient's desire for healing to Allah, who then responds back through the *rabs* to the supplicant(s).

Trances, where *the rab* inhabits a dancer, are a key feature of *Ndepp* ceremonies. The dancer begins to move in a way that is characteristic of a particular *rab*, and those movements are recognized by the *Ndeppkats* or others in the group with experience.

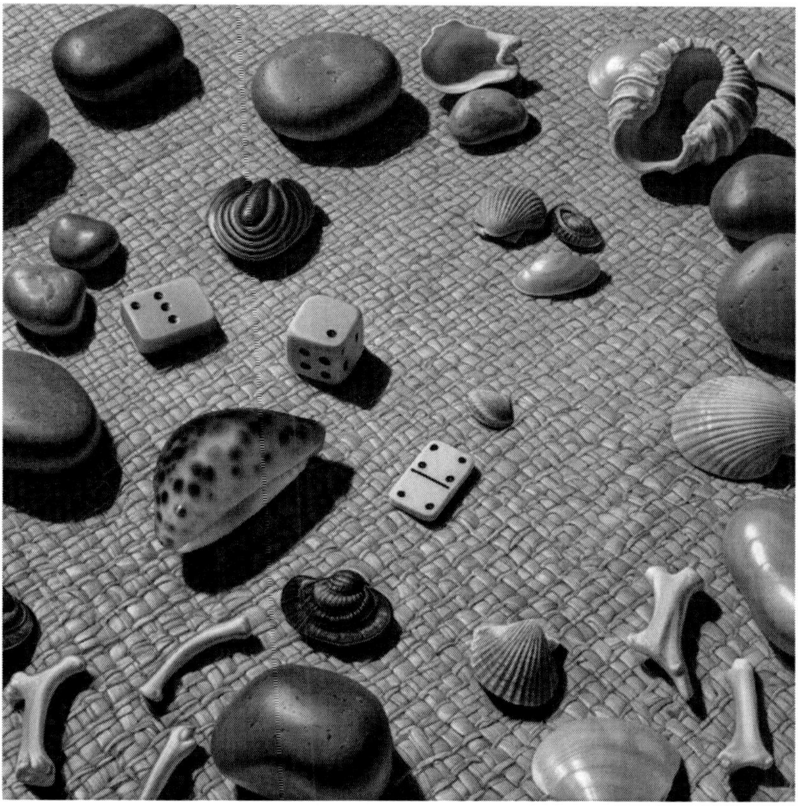

Figure 9
Sample of objects used in Swaziland for divining.

Thus, the *rab* who is going to be responsible for the healing is identified. This 'riding,' i.e., "possession" of the devotee through trance, also binds the *rab* and his/her devotee ever more closely together. The animal sacrifice will be offered if it is required. Examples of animals used are: a chicken, goat, sheep, or a bull in ascending order of power. When a bull is sacrificed, certain parts are distributed in seven sacred places. Note that the way a bull is tied for sacrifice in Ndepp is unchanged from the way it was done in ancient Egypt. What is more, the way in which the bull

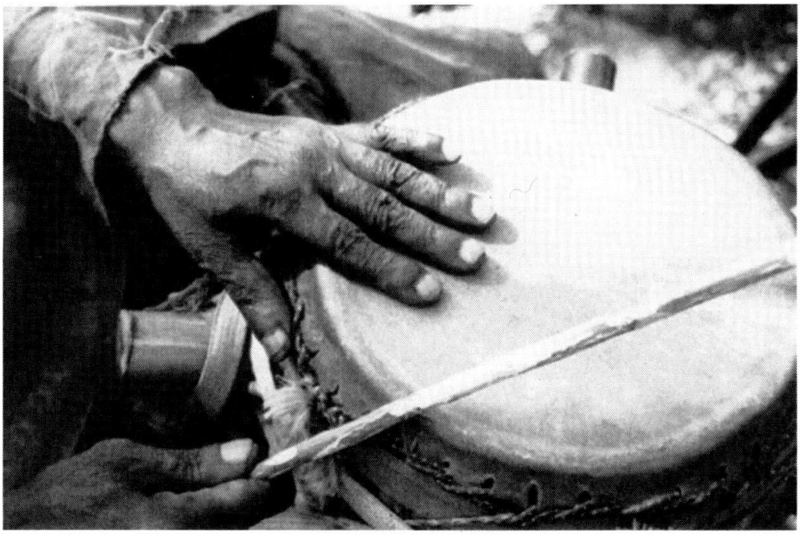

Figure 10
Hands of an Ndepp drummer. Photo by Lenny Foster.

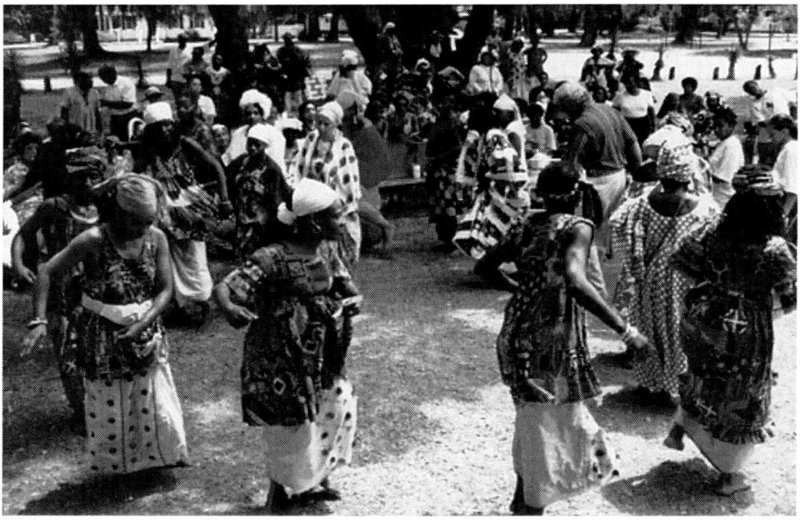

Figure 11
Circular dance in an Ndepp ceremony. Photo by Lenny Foster.

is butchered, drawn, quartered, divided up and redistributed in certain places can be seen in ritual slaughtering scenes in the temples of Egypt. The sacrifice represents an energy exchange mediated through the power of blood, the river of life. For renewed life, which is what healing is, life force is required—hence the need for sacrifice in many instances. Later, the *Ndeppkats* may offer herbs, with pharmacologic properties—but also healing energies, not measurable in biochemical terms—to the individual who is ill. Just as in modern medicine, the individual suffering the illness is given instructions, or a prescription, for continued healing. Sometimes herbal baths are required in addition to imbibing the herbal mixtures. The meat of the sacrificed animal is cooked, and the food is shared by the entire village, providing all with the benefit of the healing life force.

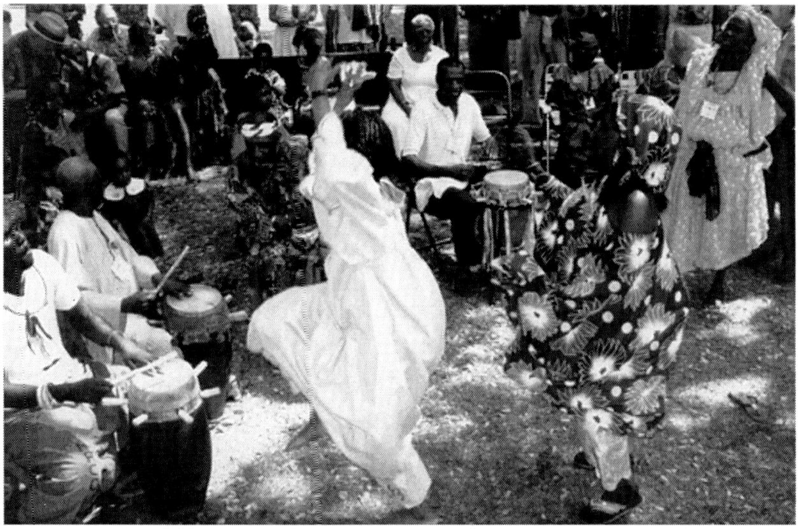

Figure 12
Drumming and dancing for spirit. **Photo by Lenny Foster.**

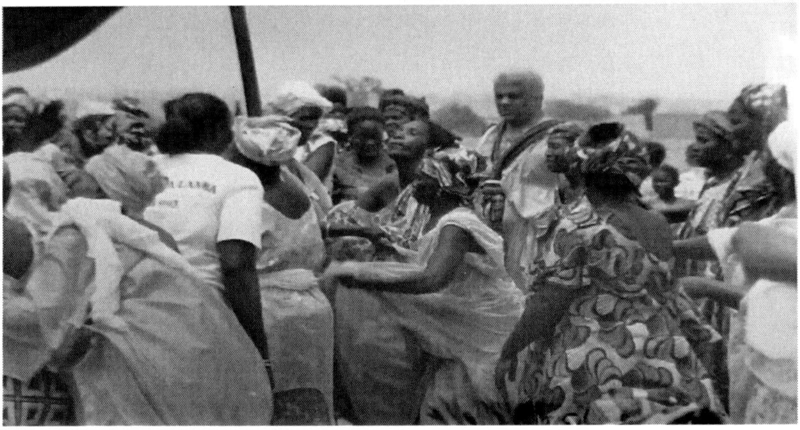

Figure 13
Coumba Lamba Ceremony. Photo by Iris Green.

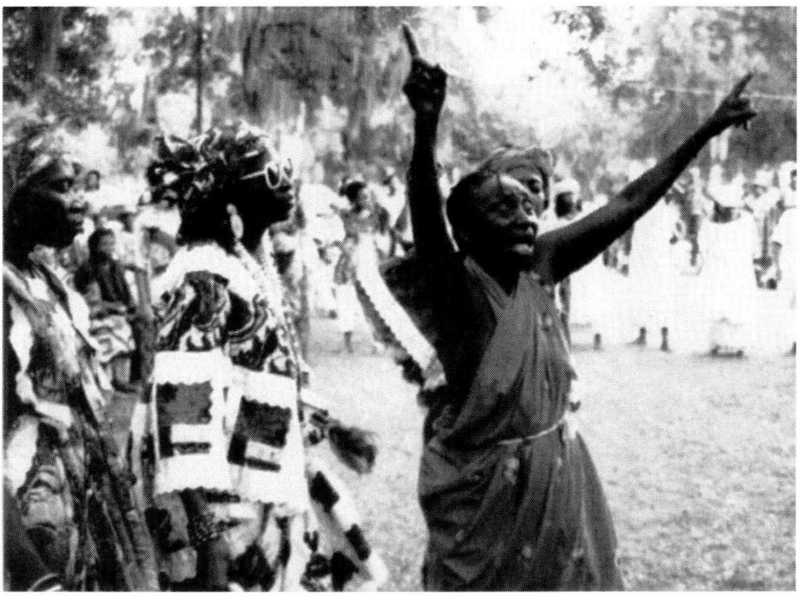

Figure 14
Descent of the Rab—Maam Massamba Ndoye. Photo by Lenny Foster.

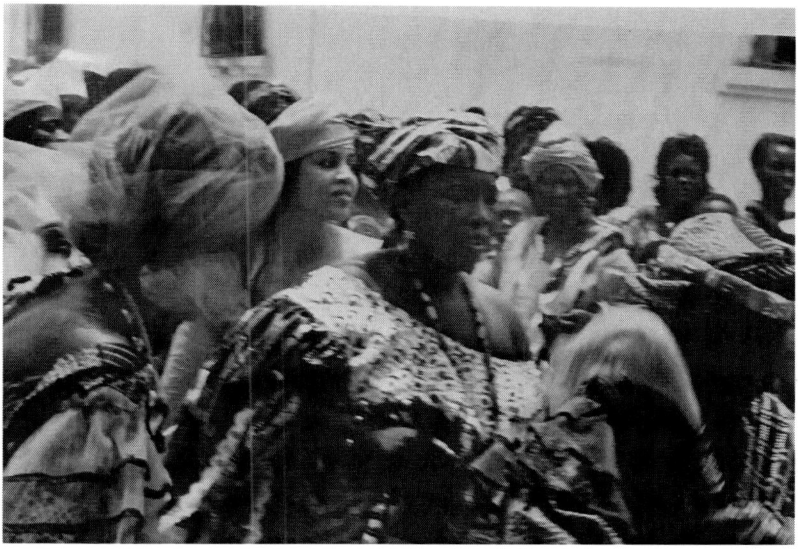

Figure 15

The Ndeppkats traveled from village to village after the Coumba Lamba ceremony doing healing dances. People came out of their dwellings to get near the dancers for healing energies. Photo by Iris Green.

Sacrifice: The Nexus of Life and Death

The evolution of human consciousness has always been mediated by the idea and practice of sacrifice. It is certainly fundamental to all mytho-religious impulses that motivate human beings, but in some sense sacrifice seems innate to the life process itself. Life, since this creation occurred 12 billion years ago, only continues through a process of becoming. Thus, while "beingness" never changes, its outward forms always do. Becoming is therefore a continuous, interactive process of organizing, disorganizing, and re-organizing. In biological terms this reveals itself as life, death, and rebirth. Life and death, therefore, are so interlocked that one defines and makes possible the other. The process of becoming, so essential to existence, depends absolutely on the interplay between life and death.

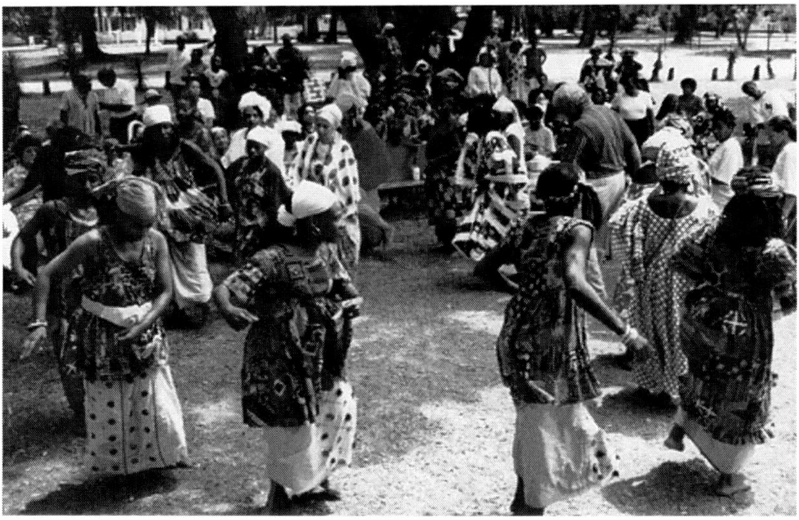

Figure 16
Circular dance in an Ndepp ceremony. **Photo by Lenny Foster.**

If we can refrain from looking at life merely as "affirmation" and death as "negation," we will be better prepared to see their interrelation as the "force of being" exchanging forms. When this vision of existence emerges, life and death each loses some of its terror. We have the idea that the "will to live," i.e., what the psychoanalysts like to call *eros*, is all-powerful, and indeed it is exceedingly strong. But there comes a time when *thanatos*, the "death instinct," overtakes *eros*; and the release from the bonds of life becomes a welcome prospect. Moreover, in traditional African thought, dying on this plane of existence means birth on another, and vice-versa. It's a dance that life and death do, and the music never stops.

With this philosophic preamble, we can begin to grasp the role, function, and significance of sacrifice. Ultimately, a sacrifice, no matter what form it takes, has the effect of strengthening the life force of one by appropriating the life force of another. It can be seen as an exchange of energy. There are, of course, ascending levels of complexity and potency. In the world of *Ndepp* of the Lebu people of Senegal, the milk sacrifice is an "entry-level" sacrifice. Since milk is expressed from the udders of a living thing, cow or goat, it embodies some of the life force of that animal.

Ascending levels of sacrificial potency in *Ndepp* move beyond the milk sacrifice into the hierarchy of blood sacrifice, starting with chickens, ascending to goats, then sheep, and finally to bulls. These are ever-larger animals, each possessing incrementally more life force than the one below it. The appropriateness of using one as opposed to another depends on the severity of the problem encountered, or the seriousness of the transformation undertaken. It is well to note that the rituals and sacrifices for healing are identical to those for initiation. A healing and an initiation both entail the "dying" of the old self and the "birth" of a new self. For the transfer to be successful, the human must bond physically, mentally, and spiritually with the animal to be sacrificed before it dies. Established rituals in the healing ceremony allow the bonding and transfer to occur.

When a blood sacrifice is called for, it means that the life potency of the victim, carried in his blood, is deemed necessary to effect transformation. As a newborn comes into life bathed in blood, so a new birth through healing or initiation recreates the same process. The initiate *ipso facto* becomes twin to the sacrificial victim; the victim becomes the other self who infuses the healed individual or the initiate with new life, and carries away the dysfunctional accretions of the old life with him. The beneficiary so renewed in this manner is deeply indebted to the victim in a manner similar to the Christian debt to Christ for his sacrificial death on the Cross. This analogy is sharpened by New Testament references to Christ as "the sacrificial lamb" who took on our sins, and whose blood washes and purifies us.

There is much sacrifice that is called for in *Ndepp* and in other indigenous systems because it is believed that we are not collectively a spiritually sound, psychologically healthy or empowered people. When ancient Kemet was in her golden age, a sacrifice of the Apis Bull was only effected once every nine years for the whole country!

Modern culture abhors the notion of animal sacrifice because of its "pagan," hence "barbaric" overtones, but is it really primitive, barbaric, or savage? If one eats meat, or even harvests plants for food, has there not been a sacrifice to put that food on the table—a sacrifice without ritual or meaning behind it in most cases? The writer remembers the first day in his college biology lab when the chief instructor gathered 200 students together to explain the initial procedures. The instructor assured us that he understood the moral reservations of some students about killing animals for the purposes of teaching and research, but said that we were to "think of it as a *sacrifice*!" Indeed, biomedical scientists routinely refer to "sacrificing an animal" when they kill it in the course of research. In any given year, millions of animals—mice, rats, hamsters, dogs, cats, monkeys, chimpanzees, etc. are "sacrificed" for scientific purposes. Thus, the modern world practices animal sacrifice on a huge scale with the justification that sacrifice is necessary for science and for food. Yet, both in African traditional ceremonies and in the Western World, sacrifice is seen as beneficial to the society, the community, and ultimately, the individual.

As Native Americans, and other indigenous peoples believe, the act of dying may be good or bad, peaceful or violent, dignified or terrifying, but in and of itself, death is not the enemy. The Lakota used to say, if there were no death, life would be without joy or meaning. Moreover, it is death that teaches us most about life. This message was conveyed by Don Juan Matus to Carlos Casteneda in the series of seven books written by Castenada on the Yaqui Way of Knowledge.[9] Such an attitude is found also in the ancient Egyptian story of "A Dialogue of a Man with his Ka."[10] Life and death form a nexus point in sacrificial ritual that continually renews our existence. It is a necessary guidepost as we traverse the often tortuous path toward spiritual wholeness

When one goes to the any of the African traditional systems with impeccable intent, one can partake of the power of these systems in such a way as to enhance life for self, family, and community. The significance of these rituals extends beyond their immediate spiritual impacts; they are deeply embedded at the very core of the human psyche as mechanisms for personal and communal healing and renewal. By examining these practices through a lens of shared humanity rather than through the bifurcated view of "us" versus "them," it becomes possible to

9 7 Books by Carlos Castaneda, New York, Pocket Books/Washington Square Press:
The Teachings of Don Juan: A Yaqui Way of Knowledge
A Separate Reality: Further Conversations with Don Juan
Journey to Ixtlan: The Lessons of Don Juan
Tales of Power
The Second Ring of Power
The Eagle's Gift
The Fire from Within
The Power of Silence

10 Also known as: *A dialog of a Man with his Ba*, Berlin Papyrus 3024.

appreciate the profound spiritual and existential questions that sacrifice poses, inviting a more inclusive exploration of its role in human history and consciousness. The discourse on sacrifice within the African context, therefore, serves not only as a reflection on the spiritual and cultural practices of African societies but also as a mirror reflecting the broader human condition, challenging us to reconsider our own views on life, death, and the rituals that define and bind our collective human experiences. Through this exploration, the author seeks to illuminate the depths of African spiritual and healing practices, providing a richer, more nuanced understanding of their significance and sophistication.

A word about the future of African traditional medicine. Since the time of Egyptians, the transfer of medical knowledge, was mostly hereditary—father to son, or mother to daughter. Teaching new practitioners was complex, involving not only didactic learning, but also dance, song, rhythm, gesture, and symbol, says Gbodossou.[11] "The elders who are the repository of traditional culture—the priests, healers, mediums, and herbalists—are dying. And young people are no longer being groomed in sufficient numbers to take their place."[12] To save traditional knowledge, some organizations have begun to support and partner with traditional healers. Modern medicine is no longer ignoring the success of traditional medicine, but instead is looking for ways to integrate it into the total plan for community health in many areas.

The author found in his study of the Serer healers at Malango (1992) that 90% of the individuals who came there for help

11 Op. sit., Gbodossou, p. 9
12 Ibid., p. 11

reported a favorable outcome to their condition.[13] Erick Gbodossou founded *PROMETRA* (Promotion des Médecines Traditionelles), which is now collaborating with the Morehouse School of Medicine. The mission of PROMETRA International is to preserve African traditional medicine, culture and indigenous science through research, education, development, advocacy and service; and to improve the health and well being of Africa and the Diaspora. The *Global Initiative for Traditional Systems of Health* (**GIFTS**) is a program launched in 1993.

The World Health Organization (WHO) has several initiatives to promote traditional medicine globally, including the WHO Global Traditional Medicine Centre (GTMC) and the WHO Traditional Medicine Global Summit. These organizations are using traditional healing methods and medicines made from native plants and trees to fight modern diseases like Ebola, HIV/AIDS and COVID-19. The WHO Traditional Medicine Strategy 2014–2023 was developed and launched in response to the World Health Assembly resolution on traditional medicine (WHA62.13). The strategy aims to support Member States in developing proactive policies and implementing action plans that will strengthen the role traditional medicine plays in keeping populations healthy.[14]

One cannot stand in judgement of traditional African practices without understanding the full meaning of a complex, holistic, communal healing process, which is, indeed, at the basis of our contemporary religious and healing philosophies.

13 Finch, C, *A knowledge, Attitudes, and Practices Survey of Traditional Healers in Fatick, Senegal*, 1992, USAID Grant #685-0281-G-00-1254-00, p. 156

14 Sixty-second World Health Assembly WHA62.13 Agenda item 12.4 22 May 2009

While we cannot deny nor condone the use of such traditions for the purpose of deliberately causing hurt or harm, we must also stand in awe of the African physician-priest's ability to work within, around and through the laws of nature, which are indeed the principles of quantum physics! Are we dealing with superstition, primitive savagery, or science of the highest order? Modern medicine is now ready to become the pupil, for there is much to be learned.

APPENDIX I

A Knowledge, Attitudes, and Practices Survey of Traditional Healers in Fatick, Senegal

1992

CHARLES S. FINCH III, M.D.

Project Funded by
UNITED STATES AGENCY FOR INTERNATIONAL DEVELOPMENT
Grant #685-0281-G-00-1254-00
The content is solely the responsibility of the author and does not necessarily represent the official views of the USAID.

I. Introduction

This report entails a detailed exposition of the recent Healers Knowledge, Attitudes, and Practices (KAP) Survey (USAID-Senegal Grant #685-0281-G-00-1254-00) in Fatick, Senegal. The preliminary report that has already been submitted described the history of the project up to the final meeting held June 27–28, 1992 at Le Centre Saidou Nourou Tall in Mbour. In this document, the relevant data will be reviewed and the applicability of this data to helping solve some of the health care problems of contemporary Senegal will be discussed. The report will be divided into four sections: (I.) Introduction, (II.) Healers Survey, (III.) Villagers Survey, and (IV.) Comment.

The data base is voluminous and not all of the information can be covered by this report. However, the salient results will be highlighted and the print-out made available for those wishing to review the figures in detail. Much information still reposes in the mass of raw data gleaned from nearly 900 questionnaires (includes the healer and village surveys) and this constitutes a valuable repository that can be mined in the future to answer other questions.

II. Healers Survey

Questionnaire

The questionnaire contained 330 separate items in nine sections. Section VI, containing 21 questions concerning the diagnosis and treatment of specific illnesses could, theoretically, be repeated 50 times because there were 50 illnesses listed in the survey. This could maximally give an additional 1,050 items. In practice, this did not occur because no healer listed more than 10 illnesses in his healing "repertoire."

All the interviews were conducted in Serer by interviewers who were bi-lingual in French and Serer and who thus transcribed all the responses onto the questionnaire in French. The numbers in parentheses next to each item listed below represent the number of valid questionnaires for each item. The percentages recorded are the **valid percentages,** that is they are computed on the basis of the number of valid questionnaires for each item.

A. *Identification Data*

1. **Interview Months:** The healer survey was carried out between December 16, 1991 and February 26, 1992. In the healers' survey, 76 or 20.2% of the questionnaires were completed in December, 178 or 47.3% were completed in January, and 122 or 32.4% were completed in February, for a total of 376 completed questionnaires. This number represents 98% of the total number of healers (383) belonging to the Healers' Association at Malango (Fatick).

2. **Reasons for Non-participation:** There were six members or 1.6% of the 383 belonging to the Healers' Association who did not participate in the survey. Two of these individuals refused outright and four do not actually practice traditional medicine.

3. **Arrondisement (District) of the Interview (375):** 93 or 24.9% of the interviews were conducted in Diakhao, 25 or 6.7% in Fatick, 95 or 25.3% in Fumela, 78 or 20.8% in Niakhar, and 83 or 22.1% in Tattaguine.

4. **Interviewer Participation (376):** There were four interviewers who conducted the survey: Coly performed 93 or 24.7% of the interviews, Dione 93 or 24.7%, Ngom 93 or 24.7%, and Sarr 97 or 25.8% of the interviews.

5. **Duration of Interview (370):** Interviews ranged from 30 minutes to 5 hours 20 minutes in length; the median duration of the interviews was 99 minutes (1 hour 39 minutes).

B. *Socio-Demographic Data*

6. **Age of the Healers (369):** Healers' ages ranged from 16 to 94 years, the median age being 59.5 years. Two hundred twenty-one (221) or 59.8% of the respondents, ranged in age from 50 to 69. It was thought initially that the preponderance of the healers toward the older end of the age scale indicated that there were few younger persons entering into this calling. This was found anecdotally to be misleading. In Serer culture, no apprentice "hangs out his shingle" until his teacher and master has died. Thus a budding healer may be apprenticed for years, even into middle age and beyond. This information did not become available until the survey was well in progress so there were no questions included to ascertain the number of active apprentices among the healers.

7. **Gender of the Healers (376):** Three hundred eleven (311) or 82.7% of the healers were men and 65 or 17.3% were women. By inter-ethnic comparison, the Lebu healing rituals of **Ndepp** are controlled mostly by women.

8. **Ethnicity (374):** Three hundred fifty-one (351) or 93.4% of the healers were ethnic Serer, 10 or 2.7% were Wolof, 8 or 2.1% were Pulaar, and the small remainder were Bambara, Sarakhole, and Moorish. These ratios are to be expected in a region where the important Serer kingdom of Sine once held sway.

9. **Changes of Residence (374):** Two hundred seventy-seven (227) or 74.1% of the respondents live and work in the village where they were born. This figure reveals a striking degree of geographic stability which, along with other indicators (see **11. Marriage),** seem to suggest that the healers

strongly represent a conservative, stabilizing force in their communities.

10. **Religion (374):** One hundred forty-seven (147) or 39.9% of the healers identified themselves as exclusively Muslim, 124 or 33.2% as a mixture of "Muslim-Animist," 40 or 10.7% as exclusively Christian, 37 or 9.9% as a mixture of "Christian-Animist," and 25 or 6.7% as purely Animists. A preferable designation for "Animist" might have been "Serer-traditional" but whatever the case, these responses indicate that traditional Serer beliefs still hold sway even among those practicing other organized religions (Islam and Christianity). This is rather the rule throughout Muslim (and Christian) Africa, where incoming religions are modified in the African pattern.

11. **Marriage:** Three hundred thirty-five (335) or 89.1% of 376 respondents were married at the time of the survey. One hundred seventy-eight (178) or 47.8% of 372 respondents had one spouse, 100 or 26.9% had two spouses, 32 or 8.6% had three spouses, 18 or 4.8% had four spouses. Of the 38 of **372** respondents that were not married at the time of the survey, 36 or 94.7% were widowed. Though there are no figures on re-marriage after divorce, these data would still seem to indicate a high level of domestic stability among the healers.

12. **Children (374):** Three hundred sixty-two (362) or 96.8% of the respondents reported having living children, though 277 or 74% of them have lost at least one child.

13. **Principal Occupation (361):** Only 43 or 11.9% of the respondents practice traditional medicine as their principal

occupation. Two hundred ninety-seven (297) or 82.3% of them practice agriculture, with or without livestock raising, as their principal occupation. Thus only a small minority of the healers can make a living exclusively as practitioners.

C. *Work Habits of the Healers*

14. **Days per Week of Practice (371) and Numbers of Patients Seen (359):** Three hundred five (305) or 82.2% of **371** respondents indicated that they see patients six or seven days per week. Two hundred fifty-nine (259) or 72.1% of **359** respondents reported having seen between one and seven patients in the week immediately preceding the interview. Eighty-two (82) or 22.8% of **359** reported having seen no patients in the week preceding the interview, 26 or 7.2% reported having seen 10 patients, and two respondents reported seeing 50 patients in the week preceding the interview.

15. **Conditions Under Which the Healer Will Call on the Patient (371):** One hundred eighty-six (186) or 50.1% of the respondents reported visiting the patient to treat a problem. Of these **186** respondents, 181 or 97.3% make "house calls" upon request of the patient or patient's family; one hundred thirty-two (132) or 70.9% of these **186** do so by appointment.

16. **Treatment "Prerequisites":** Two hundred fifty-two (252) of **353** or 71.3% of the respondents required payment in advance for treatment. Ninety-one (91) of **352** or 25.8% of the respondents indicated that financial support from the client's family was required for certain treatments. One

hundred forty-two (142) of **353** or 40.2% responded that the husband's presence was required for the treatment of married women and 102 of **350** or 29.1% responded that the husband's permission, with or without his presence, was sufficient to treat married women.

17. **Work at Malango Center (372):** Only 78 or 21% of the respondents work at the Malango Center, a traditional healing clinic in Fatick affiliated with the Traditional Healers' Association. Largely this is due to limited facilities that can only accomodate 10–15 healers on a given day. The Malango Center operates seven days a week and at least four of the healers reside there permanently. Since opening formally in February, 1989, nearly 5,000 patients have been seen there.

18. **Membership in the Healers' Association (366):** One hundred forty (140) or 38.3% of the respondents reported having belonged to the Association since its inception (circa 1975); 115 or 31.4% reported having joined within the 12 months prior to the time of the interview.

19. **Attitude Toward the Association (331):** Three hundred thirteen (313) or 94.5% report deriving some benefit from their membership in the Association; 16 or 4.8% deny any benefit from membership.

20. **Motives for Membership in the Association (326):** Ninety-seven or 29.8% of the respondents desire collaboration with other healers, 63 or 19.3% feel they are serving their country by their membership, 47 or 14.4% wish to revive traditional medicine, and 36 or 11% cite the opportunity to exchange knowledge.

21. **Consultation of Other Healers (372):** One Hundred thirty-six (136) or 36.5% of the respondents reported consulting with other healers. Of these **136** respondents, 84 or 61.8% cited the desire to improve their knowledge as a reason for consulting other healers, 26 or 19.1% cited their inability to handle specific cases, 14 or 10.3% cited the need to collaborate on complicated cases, and 4 or 2.9% reported that certain of their colleagues were known to be successful specialists for certain problems.

D. *Education and Training of the Healers*

22. **French Schooling (374):** Only 27 or 7.2% of the respondents had French education to any level.

23. **French Language Capability (373):** Just 26 or 7% of the respondents speak French, 23 or 6.2% read French, and 19 or 5.1% write French.

24. **Koranic Schooling (374):** Only 18 or 4.8% of the respondents attended Koranic school.

25. **Arabic Language Capability (374):** Just 5 or 1.3% of the respondents speak Arabic, 9 or 2.4% read Arabic, and 7 or 1.9% write Arabic. As seen above **(10. Religion),** nearly 40% of the healers are exclusively Muslim and may be presumed to recite some of their prayers in Arabic. If this is the case, it must be concluded that the prayers were learned by rote.

26. **Native Language (374):** The native language is Serer for 353 or 94.4% of the respondents. The next largest native language category is Wolof for 10 or 2.7% of the respon-

dents. Three hundred forty-four (344) of **368** (93.5%) of the respondents use Serer as their "language of work."

27. **Second Language (344):** Three hundred twenty-two (322) or 93.6% of the respondents speak Wolof. Wolof is the national language of Senegal, spoken by more than 90% of the population, regardless of ethnicity.

28. **The Means of Becoming a Healer (373):** In this item, there is an overlapping of the categories of responses, that is to say that there is usually more than one means by which the budding healer is given access to healing knowledge. Three hundred twenty-nine (329) or 88.2% of the respondents reported inheriting their knowledge from an older family member, usually a parent. Thus traditional healing tends to be a family occupation handed down from generation to generation. Three hundred twenty-six (326) or 87.4% reported receiving their training by apprenticeship, whether as a family inheritance or not. As seen above **(6. Age of the Healers),** an apprenticeship can last many years. As indicated, a significant minority of apprentices (20%) can and do come from outside the family circle.

    Two hundred eleven (211) or 56.6% of the respondents reported receiving their healing knowledge as "a gift of the **pangools,"** who are the Serer ancestral and cosmic spirits that rule their universe. This is consistent with their reports that much of their healing knowledge—both empirical and ritualistic—comes to them in dreams. Related to this is the report of 89 or 23.9% of them that their knowledge comes to them as a "gift of God." As mentioned above, none of these categories is mutually exclusive so that a given healer may receive knowledge by one or more means more or less seamlessly at the same time.

29. **Inheritance of Healing Vocation (373):** One hundred fifty-eight (15 8) or 42.4% of the respondents reported inheriting their healing vocation through their maternal lineage whereas 261 or 70% reported inheriting through their paternal lineage. These numbers indicate that a significant number of healers inherit their healing vocation through both lineages.

30. **Healing Vocation by Apprenticeship (373):** One hundred twenty-seven (127) or 34% of the respondents reported apprenticing themselves to teachers in their maternal lineage, 225 or 60.3% reported apprenticing themselves to teachers in their paternal lineage, 70 or 18.8% reported apprenticing themselves to healers who had cured them, and 78 or 20.9% reported apprenticing themselves to healers who had cured a member of their family. The apparent discrepancy between these numbers vis-a-vis lineage and those in item **#29 (Inheritance of Healing Vocation)** can be explained by inheritance of the healing vocation sometimes being passed on not by apprenticeship but by direct spiritual intervention (See **31. Healing Knowledge as a Gift of the Spirits** below).

31. **Healing Knowledge as a Gift of the Spirits*** **(373):** Two hundred eight (208) or 55.8% of the respondents reported receiving their knowledge from the spirits **(pangools)** through dreams. Twenty-nine (29) or 7.8% reported being taught directly by a **Djinn,** a Muslim elemental spirit, and 41 or 11% report receiving their knowledge from a **dwarf,** a special category of being said to possess extraordinary powers.

*See Appendix for definition of these terms.

32. **Age at Beginning of Training (351):** The age range for beginning training spanned ages four (4) to seventy-four (74) years, with the median age being 19.5 years.

33. **Duration of Training (341):** The range of duration of training spanned less-than-one-year to 64 years with the median duration being 14.5 years.

34. **By Whom or through What Means Was Training Conducted (369):*** Three hundred fourteen (314) or 85% of the respondents reported instruction by a herbalist, 63 or 17% reported instruction by a **louloup,** 59 or 15.9% reported instruction by a **saltigue (guerisseur** or **elu),** 178 or 48.2% reported instruction by a **yaal pangool,** and 103 or 27.9% reported learning through various divination or clairvoyant methods, i.e., **cowries, sand, palm reading,** and **water.**

*See Appendix for definition of these terms.

35. **Disciplines in Which Healers Were Trained (376):** Three hundred fifty (350) or 93% of the respondents reported learning the application of medicinal plants, 340 or 90.3% reported learning methods of incantation, 308 or 81.8% reported learning how to prescribe special foods and beverages, 289 or 76.8% reported learning how to use "other natural products," 285 or 75.7% reported learning the application of vaporous inhalations, 285 or 75.7% reported learning how to prescribe special baths, 226 or 60.1% reported learning the usage of various animal products, 190 or 50.5% reported learning massage techniques, 136 or 36.1% reported learning how to divine by clairvoyant methods, and 115 or 30.5%

reported learning how to "treat at a distance." It is also noteworthy that 24 or 6.3% learned how to set bones.

E. *Services Provided by the Healers*

36. **Therapeutic specialties (376):*** Three hundred fifty (350) or 93% of the respondents classify themselves as **herbalists,** 167 or 44.4% classify themselves as **yaal pangool,** 59 or 15.7% classify themselves as **louloups,** 190 or 50.5% classify themselves as **clairvoyants** by incantation, sand, or cowry methods. There are other classifications under the category of **clairvoyant** but those listed here represent more than 90% of them. These numbers show that healers may be adept in more than one specialty.

*See Appendix for definition of the categories discussed under this item.

37. **The Purpose of Clairvoyance (372):** One hundred thirty-three (133) or 35.7% of the respondents reported using clairvoyant methods to predict the future, 144 or 38.7% reported using them to make a diagnosis for their patients, 106 or 28.4% reported using them to determine the plants needed for treating a particular disorder, and 151 or 40.6% reported using them to determine the nature of and the solution to psycho-social problems the client may present with.

38. **Techniques of Clairvoyance:** Two hundred nineteen (219) or 85.5% of **256** respondents reported experiencing clairvoyant dreams in their work, 38 or 28.8% of **132** respondents reported using sand divination, 8 or 10.2% of **78** respondents reported using cowry shells.

39. **Empirical Diagnostic Techniques (376):** Two hundred seventy-one (271) or 72% of the respondents reported examing the tongue of patients, 225 or 60% reported palpating the patient, 143 or 38% reported observing the patient's manner of walking, and 123 or 32.7% reported asking the patient questions concerning the nature of the illness.

F. ***Patients Consulting The Healers***

40. **Gender of Last Patient Seen (356):** One hundred seventy-one (171) or 48% of the respondents reported that their last patient was male and 185 or 52% reported that their last patient was female.

41. **(Estimated) Age of Last Patient Seen (329):** The age range of the last patient see was between under-one-year to 70 years with the median age at 29.5 years. Of all decades, the 30–39 age segment had the highest number, i.e., 82 or 24.9%. All of these age determinations must be considered approximations.

42. **Where the Last Patient Came From? (355):** One hundred thirty-eight (138) or 38.9% of the respondents reported that their last patient came from their own village, 109 or 30.7% reported that the patient came from the same arrondissement (district), 35 or 9.9% reported that the last patient came from the same departement ("county"), and 69 or 19.4% of the respondents reported that their last patient came from outside the region altogether.

43. **Who Accompanied the Last Patient? (353):** Two hundred sixteen (216) or 61.2% of the respondents reported that the

patient came alone, 56 or 15.9% reported that the patient was brought by the mother, 17 or 4.8% reported that the patient was brought by the father, 12 or 3.4% reported that the patient was brought by the husband. Forty-one (41) or 11.6% of the respondents reported that their last patient was brought by other assorted family members. It can be inferred that in most instances where a parent accompanied the patient, patient was a child or "pre-adult."

44. **Who Made the Decision to Consult the Healer? (350):** Two hundred twenty-two (222) or 63.4% of the respondents reported that the patient made the decision to come for the consultation, 56 or 16% reported that the mother made the decision, 22 or 6.3% reported that the father made the decision, and 15 or 4.3% reported that the husband made the decision. As in item no. 43, most of the parental decisions involving the consultation with the healer probably involved children or pre-adults.

45. **Was the Healer Recommended to the Patient? (356):** One hundred fifty-nine (159) or 44.7% of the respondents reported that some one had specifically recommended the healer to the last patient for the problem under consultation whereas 197 or 55.3% denied it.

46. **Who Recommended the Healer to the Patient? (152):** Forty-five (45) or 29.6% of the respondents (answered item no. 45 in the affirmative) reported that some one who knew the healer by name (and presumably reputation) had recommended their last patient, 35 or 23% reported that a former patient (cured) had made the recommendation, 16 or 10.5% reported that the person accompanying their last

patient had made the recommendation, 13 or 8.6% reported that some one in the healer's own family had made the recommendation, 10 or 6.6% reported that it was a relative of the patient that had made the recommendation.

47. **Method of Payment of the Last Patient (356):** Just nine (9) or 2.5% of the respondents reported being paid in kind, 304 or 85.4% reported being paid in cash, 28 or 7.9% reported not being paid at all (16 or 4.5% of these were due to the indigence of the patient), and 10 or 2.8% reported that the results of the cure are being awaited before payment is given. Anecdotally, it is known that among the clientele of the traditional healers, the payment is considered part of the healing process which helps account for a payment rate approaching 90%.

48. **Follow-up of Patients (351):** Three hundred thirty-eight (338) or 96.3% of the respondents reported that they followed up on their patients whereas 13 or 3.7% denied it.

49. **Methods of Follow-up (338):** Sixty-five (65) or 19.2% of the respondents reported that the patients returned to them in the course of the cure, 112 or 33.1% reported that the patients came back to express their thanks for a successful cure, 32 or 9.5% reported that they were in daily (permanent) contact with the patient, 36 or 10.7% reported that the patients were required to return to give an account of the progress of the cure, 34 or 10% reported that some of their patients had regular return appointments, and 13 or 3.5% reported that contact with **pangools** (spirits) allowed them to keep informed about their patients.

G. *Illnesses Treated by the Healers*

50. **List of Number of Percentage:** Based on No. of Respondents in ()

List of Illnesses	Number of Healers	Percentage: Based on No. of Respondents in ( )
Sexually Transmitted Disease	129	35.0% (369)
Migraine	110	29.8% (369)
Diarrhea	101	27.4% (369)
Labor & Delivery	93	25.3% (368)
Feminine Sterility	85	23.0% (369)
Parasitosis	83	22.6% (368)
Yellow Fever	79	21.5% (368)
Hemorrhoids	78	21.2% (368)
Contraception	71	19.2% (369)
Impotence	63	17.1% (369)
Wound Treatment	62	16.8% (370)
Abnormal Uterine Bleeding	56	15.1% (370)
Malaria	55	14.9% (368)
Abortion	52	14.1% (369)
Meningitis	28	7.6% (368)
Tonsillitis	46	12.5% (368)
Bronchitis	44	12.0% (368)
Dental Problems	44	11.9% (369)
Heart Attack	42	11.4% (369)
Skin Eruptions	41	11.1% (368)
Snake-bite	39	10.6% (369)
Tetanus	38	10.3% (368)
Epilepsy	38	10.3% (368)
Mental Illness	37	10.0% (369)
G.I. Ulcers	36	9.8% (368)

List of Illnesses	Number of Healers	Percentage: Based on No. of Respondents in ( )
Hepatitis	35	9.5% (368)
Kidney Disease	35	9.5% (368)
Ear Infection	35	9.5% (368)
Hernia	35	9.5% (369)
Gastrointestinal Bleeding	34	9.2% (368)
Measles	34	9.2% (368)
Prostate Disorders	34	9.2% (369)
Uterine Prolapse	34	9.2% (369)
Tuberculosis	30	8.2% (368)
Asthma	30	8.2% (368)
Tumors/Cancer	29	7.9% (368)
Leprosy	29	7.9% (368)
Meningitis	28	7.6% (368)
Hypertension	27	7.3% (368)
Diabetes	25	6.8% (368)
Stroke	25	6.8% (368)
Fractures/Dislocations	24	6.5% (369)
Burns	24	6.5% (369)
Goiter	21	5.7% (368)
Sinusitis	19	5.2% (368)

There were numerous other illnesses (44) mentioned by the healers that are not listed here. The most common of these (mentioned by at least 5% of the healers) were **mauvais vent*** ("ill wind"), eye disorders, and rheumatism.

*See Appendix for definition of these terms.

51. **Etiology-Spiritual (301):** One hundred ninety-five (195) or 64.7% of the respondents reported various spiritual or

non-physicial factors as the principal cause of disease. These can include **seytane*, mauvais vent*,** mystical problems generally, bad spirits, and God. Generally a spiritual etiology is brought on by some social, ethical, familial, or ritual transgression that offends a higher being. These may be "sins" of omission or commission.

*See Appendix for definition of these terms.

52. **Etiology-Natural (363):** Two hundred twenty-four or 61.7% of the respondents affirmed that there are exclusively natural causes for certain diseases. For example, 122 of **269** (45.5%) healers affirmed that malaria is caused by mosquitos and 177 of **247** (71.7%) affirmed that skin eruptions have a natural etiology including poor hygiene, impurity of the blood, or internal maladies.

H. *Concepts of Anatomy and Physiology*

The majority of the healers did not supply answers to this section and it can reliably be inferred that such anatomico-physiological knowledge is largely lacking. Nonetheless there were certain categories of answers that were very revealing under each sub-heading (the number of responses are given in parentheses). Philosophical or symbolic ideas blend seamlessly with "empirical" notions.

Substantial anatomico-physiological knowledge existed in past ages in Africa and what is reported below may be a remnant of such knowledge. On the other hand, it may represent the fruit of observation and reflection by individual healers.

53. The Brain:

a. The milieu that guides man's reflection (21).
b. It is the "all" of man (7).
c. The brain controls the individual; if the brain is attacked, the person becomes depressed and is unable to control himself (4).
d. It is the center of the human being (12).
e. Without the brain there is madness(22). The brain is consciousness (2).
f. It controls individual intelligence (35).
g. The brain keeps the person in equilibrium (7).
h. It is the command center of individual (30).

54. The Kidneys:

a. The kidneys support the vessels.
b. Assure procreation (4).
c. Support the inferior parts of the body (8).
d. Constitute a vital part of the organism (7).
e. They are the relay points between the upper and lower halves of the body (9).
f. They contain the "current" and good humor of the individual.
g. The kidneys are the center of man's physical strength (8).

55. The Heart:

a. An individual's life depends on the functioning of the heart (4).
b. If the heart stops beating, the person dies (2).
c. The heart is the seat of courage (27).

d. The heart is almost like the brain (2). It represents the "soul" of individual (2).
e. It plays a crucial role in the organism (9).
f. It irrigates and moistens the body (and pumps) the blood (37).
g. It is the center of a person's temperment (3).
h. It supplies the organism with fluid.
i. It is the repository of individual temperment (3).
j. It modifies and regulates the person (17).

56. Stomach and Intestines

a. Storehouse of food (85).
b. Food pouches assuring digestion; grind [food] (52).
c. The stomach stores the food and the intestines move it forward and evacuate it (23).

57. Lungs:

a. Air sacks for breathing (43).
b. Assure the entrance and exit of air into the organism (11).
c. It is an organ indispensible for life (11).
d. They purify the blood originating from the heart.
e. They play a role in common with and complementary to the heart (10).

58. Reproductive Organs:

a. For conception to birth (70).
b. Permits men and women to reproduce (96).
c. They permit conjugal relations for pleasure (28); without these organs life would have no meaning (12).

d. Sustains proliferation of the species; without women, a man could live to at least 100 years.

e. They serve the same function as the kidneys: procreation (4).

I. *Relations Between Modern and Traditional Medicine*

59. Nearest Modern Health Care Facility/Personnel (373): There were six categories listed in the questionnaire but it is perhaps indicative of the status of modern health care delivery in Senegal that not one of the respondents lived within 20 kilometers of a pharmacy or clinic, much less a full-fledged hospital. The closest modern health facility was a dispensary for 275 or 73.7% of the respondents, a health outpost **(case de sante)** for 94 or 25.2% of the respondents, and a trained mid-wife for 4 or 1.1% of the respondents.

60. Referral to Modern Health Facility (372): One hundred thirty-two (132) or 35.5% of the respondents reported referring patients to a modern health care facility and 240 or 64.5% denied doing so.

61. Problems for Which at Least 5% of Referring Healers Sent Patients to a Modern Health Facility (132): Of the healers that sent patients to the modern health facility, 66 or 50% sent patients with malaria, 17 or 12.9% sent patients with dysentery, 11 or 8.3% sent laboring mothers, 8 or 6.1% sent patients with abdominal complaints, and 7 or 5.3% sent patients with open wounds.

62. **Outcome of the Last Referral to a Modern Health Facility (125):** One hundred thirteen (113) or 90.4% of the respondents reported a beneficial outcome for patients sent to a modern health facility and just 8 or 6.4% reported a negative outcome.

63. **Referral by Modern Health Practitioners to the Healers (370):** Just 40 or 10.6% of the respondents reported receiving patients by referral from a modern health facility whereas 330 or 89.2% denied any referrals from a modern health facility. Of those positively reporting referrals, five were for labor and delivery, four were for fractures, and three were for snake-bite. There were also referrals (two each) for **mauvais vent,*** **naques/seytane,*** and **anthropophagie*** ("soul-eating"). With regard to the most recent referrals, 37 of **38** respondents reported a good outcome.

*See Appendix for definition of these terms.

64. **Collaborative Work With Modern Health Practitioners (370):** Twenty-one (21) or 5.7% of the respondents reported working on a case with a modern health care practitioner whereas 349 or 94.3% of the respondents denied such collaboration.

65. **Utilization of Modern Medical Modalities (369):** Sixty-two (62) or 16.8% of the respondents reported using modern medical modalities; 307 or 83.2% denied it. Fifty-five (55) of **61** respondents utilize pharmaceutical tablets/pills and 21 of **61** administer injections.

66. **Efficacy of Modern Medicine (370):** Two hundred thirty-one (231) or 62.4% of the respondents reported that modern medicine is generally effective in curing illness whereas 139

or 37.6% reported that it is occasionally effective. No one denied the efficacy of modern medicine altogether.

67. **Perception of the Healers of Modern Practitioners' Attitudes Towards Them (373):** Two hundred forty-eight (248) or 66.5% of the respondents reported that they **do not know** modern practitioners' view of them, 53 or 14.2% reported that modern practitioners have a generally positive attitude toward healers, 11 or 2.9% reported that the attitude of modern practitioners was generally sceptical, and 60 or 16.1% reported that modern practitioners acknowledge the effectiveness of traditional medicine for certain illnesses.

68. **Separation Between Traditional and Modern Medicine (372):** Two hundred ninety-one (291) or 78.2% of the respondents reported that traditional and modern medicine are separate and distinct, 67 or 18% reported that they are not separate (are comparable).

69. **Reasons for Separateness of Traditional and Modern Medicine (292):** Two hundred twenty-seven (227) or 77.7% of the respondents reported that the practices of the two types of medicine are different, 13 or 4.5% reported that their origins were different, 13 or 4.5% reported that their belief systems are different, and 16 or 5.5% reported that their treatment modalities are different.

70. **Reasons for the Comparability of Traditional and Modern (72):** Thirty-nine (39) or 54.2% of the respondents reported that the two medical systems have the same objective, 13 or 18.1% reported that the two systems complement one another, 9 or 12.5% reported that both systems used plants. This last response may admit of several interpretations: (1)

the respondents assume, without truly knowing, that modern health care practitioners use plants in the same way healers do, (2) some modern practitioners actually do use medicinal plants under certain circumstances, or (3) this may be an oblique reference to the origin of many modern pharmaceuticals from traditional medicinal plants.

III. Village Survey

Questionnaire

The village questionnaire was devised in February immediately following the mid-project meeting. Unlike the healers' survey where no sampling was required, it was necessary to obtain a sample of villagers from the entire region of Fatick. In order to reduce sampling error to a minimum, we wanted to recruit 500 persons from 40 villages in the region for the study. We ended with 502 persons—491 actual interviews—from 29 villages, sufficiently representative to yield an acceptable sampling error. The sampling method used to obtain the study population of villagers is attached (Appendix 2).

This was a client utilization survey, the survey instrument eventually containing 81 items, about one-fourth the size of the healers' instrument. It was known from the outset that client data was necessary to provide a more complete picture of the utilization and efficacy of traditional medicine in this region. If nothing else, the client data served as a valuable cross-check of certain facets of the healer data. Early attempts to put together a qualitative client study using focus groups, key informants, etc. were abandoned because of constraints of time, funds, and appropriate resource personnel. The present survey is a modified quantitative survey.

J. *Identification Data*

71. Interview Months (502): Four hundred forty (440) or 87.6% of the interviews were conducted in the month of March and 62 or 12.4% were conducted in the month of April.

72. Arrondisements of the Study (502): One hundred fifty-five (155) or 30.9% of the villagers recruited for the study lived in Tattaguine, 111 or 22.1% lived in Diakho, 94 or 18.7% lived in Niakhar, 90 or 17.9% lived in Fumela, and 52 or 10.4% lived in Fatick.

73. Interviewer Participation (502): Coly had 129 or 25.7% interview encounters, Dione had 128 or 25.5%, Sarr 125 or 24.9%, and Ngom 120 or 23.9%

74. Completion of the Interviews (502): Four hundred ninety-one (491) or 97.8% interviews were completed with the villagers and 11 or 2.2% weren't. Of the 11 interviews not completed, one was due to a refusal and 10 were due to the absence of the interviewee.

75. Duration of the Interview (483): Interviews ranged from 10 to 67 minutes with a median duration of 20.5 minutes. The statistical mode was 20 minutes which was the length of 164 (34%) interviews.

K. *Socio-Demographic Data*

76. Age of the Villagers (485): The villagers ranged in age from 20 to 91 years with a median age of 44.5 years.

77. Gender of the Villagers (492): Two hundred forty-nine or 50.6% of the villagers were women and 243 or 49.4%

were men. A conscious effort was made during the sampling to get a statistically even gender division. The data for this report was not stratified by gender but that information is available in the data base.

78. **Ethnicity of the Villagers (491):** Four hundred eight (408) or 83.1% of the respondents identified themselves as Serer, 32 or 6.5% as Halpoular (Peul), 22 or 4.5% as Bambara, and 21 or 4.3% as Wolof. Eight of the remainder identified themselves variously as Diola, Laobe, Sarakhole, and Mandingue (Mandinke). Though, the vast majority of the population in this region is Serer, as these numbers show, there is greater diversity within the village population than among the healers themselves (94% Serer).

79. **Changes in Residence (490):** Two hundred eighty (280) or 57.1% of the respondents live in the village or district in which they were born whereas 210 or 42.9% have moved from their natal village or district. Of these respondents, 287 or 58.6% of the women and but 130 or 26.6% of the men had moved from their place of birth. Since among the Serer, patrilocal marriage patterns are dominant, about the same number of male villagers and healers (80% of whom are male) still live in their place of birth. The female villagers move more often because they go live in their husband's village after marriage.

80. **Religion (491):** Four hundred eleven (411) or 83.7% of the respondents described themselves as exclusively Muslim, 48 or 9.8% described themselves as exclusively Christian, 22 or 4.5% described themselves as Muslim-Animist, 8 or 1.9% described themselves as Christian-Animist, and 2 or

0.5% described themselves as Animist. Clearly, there has been a wholesale conversion to Islam among the villagers, much more so than found among the healers themselves. This is another datum suggesting that the healers represent a conservative force, more apt to cling to traditional ways than the general population.

81. **Marriage (491):** Three hundred ninety-nine (399) or 81.3% of the respondents were married at the time of the survey; 92 or 18.7% were not. Three hundred twenty-six (326) or 66.8% of **388** respondents reported having one spouse, 52 or 10.7% two spouses, 14 or 2.9% three spouses, and 4 or 1.6% four spouses. We can reliably infer that all of the 74 respondents that reported being married to more than one spouse were men and these 74 represented 30.4% of the village men who completed interviews (243). This compares to 50% of the sub-cohort of male healers with more than one spouse. To a large extent, this discrepancy can be explained by the difference in median age between the healer cohort and the village cohort (59.5 years vs. 44.5 years). In traditional Serer society, the ability to marry, certainly the ability to marry more than one wife, depends on a man's economic circumstances. Older men tend to be economically more established and therefore better situated to support more than one household.

There were **92** villagers who reported not being married and of these, 36 or 39.1% had never been married, 55 or 59.8% were widowed, and 1 or 1.1% were divorced. The relatively high proportion of "never-marrieds" is also undoubtedly related to the age differential of the two cohorts (healer vs. village). There were 89 respondents in the village cohort who were under age 30.

82. Children (491): Four hundred thirty-one (431) or 87.8% of the respondents reported having at least one living child. Two hundred thirty-three (233) or 47.5% of the respondents reported having at least one male child die and 221 or 45% reported having at least one female child die.

83. Principal Occupation of the Villagers (489): Two hundred two (202) or 41.3% of the respondents reported that their principal occupation was home-making. These respondents are all women and therefore represent 81.1% of the women in the cohort (249). Two hundred three (203) or 41.5% of the respondents reported that their principal occupation was agriculture with or without livestock-raising. It can be presumed that virtually all these respondents were men, representing more than 83.5% of the men in the cohort who practice agriculture as their principal means of livelihood. This compares with 82.3% of the healers (see **13. Principal Occupation)** who practice agriculture. Nineteen or 3.9% of the respondents identified themselves as artisans and 15 or 3.1% identified themselves as merchants.

L. *Education and Training of the Villagers*

84. French Schooling (491): Sixty-three or 12.8% of the respondents had spent some time in a French school. Thirty-eight (38) or 61.3% of **62** of those who had attended a French school passed through the primary level, 15 or 24.2% of them passed through the 1st secondary level, 7 or 11.3% of them passed through the 2nd secondary level, and 2 or 3.2% of them had matriculated at the university. This represents a significantly greater level of French education than the healers.

85. **French Language Capability (491):** Sixty-five or 13.2% of the villagers speak French, 63 or 12.8% read French, and 61 or 12.4% write French.

86. **Koranic Schooling (491):** Sixty-eight or 13.8% of the respondents attended Koranic school. This level of Koranic education is also significantly higher among the villagers than the healers.

87. **Arabic Language Capability (491):** 296 or 60.3% of the respondents can recite at least some of their prayers in Arabic, 25 or 5.1% can read Arabic, and 24 or 4.9% can write in Arabic.

88. **Native Language (491):** Four hundred seven (407) or 82.9% of the respondents identified themselves as native Serer-speakers, 31 or 6.3% identified themselves as Poular-speakers, 24 or 4.9% identified themselves as Bambara-speakers, and 21 or 4.3% indentified themselves as Wolof-speakers. Again, this reflects a greater degree of ethnic diversity among the villagers than among the healers. Three hundred eighty-seven or 79% of **490** of the respondents reported that they use Serer as their "every-day" language.

89. **Second Language (491):** Four hundred fifty-one or 91.9% of the respondents speak Wolof which, as noted above, is the national language of Senegal across all ethnic groups. That there are more Wolof-speakers than Serer-speakers is another indicator of the greater ethnic diversity among the villagers in the region compared to the healers. This is to say that Wolof

would be the second language for the overwhelming majority of Serer and for the other ethnic groups, meaning that there are actually more Wolof-speakers than Serer-speakers.

M. *Utilization of the Traditional Practitioner*

90. Frequency of Consultation (491): Three hundred thirty-eight (338) or 68.8% of the respondents reported that they sometimes consult traditional healers, 75 or 15.3% reported that they always consult traditional healers, 11 or 2.2% reported that they rarely consult traditional healers, and 67 or 13.6% reported that they never consult traditional healers. Thus we find that 86.4% of the villagers consult traditional healers to a greater or lesser degree, 84.1% more than rarely. This is consistent with other studies which suggest that 80% of the population throughout sub-Saharan Africa still consults traditional healers.

91. Location of the Last Consultation (421): Two hundred forty-eight (248) or 58.9% of the respondents reported that their last consultation with a traditional healer occurred in the village of the traditional healer, 164 or 39% reported that it occurred in the home of the villager, and just 9 or 2.1% reported that the last consultation took place at Malango. These latter figures seem to be rather small for Malango but since they refer only to the last consultation and since a significant percentage of the patients who consult at Malango come from outside the region, these village responses do not seem to accurately reflect the numbers of clients who consult at Malango.

92. Problem for Which the Last Consultation With the Healer Was Undertaken by at Least Five Individuals (412):

Problem	Number of Patients	Valid Percentage
Headache & Dizzyness	43	10.4%
Divination Reading	40	9.7%
Mauvais Vent	39	9.5%
Stomachache	36	8.7%
Purification	33	8.0%
Fever	21	5.1%
Mystical/Supernatural Disturbance **(Pangools)**	21	5.1%
Aches and Pains	15	3.6%
Chest Pains	12	2.9%
Side/Rib Pains	11	2.7%
Kidney Disorders	10	2.4%
General Fatigue	10	2.4%
Hernia	8	1.9%
Hemorrhoids	8	1.9%
Dermatosis	7	1.7%
Parasitosis	7	1.7%
Diarrhea	6	1.5%
Leg Pain	5	1.2%
Sore Eyes	5	1.2%
Wounds/Open Sores	5	1.2%

There were 58 different problems named by the village respondents as the motivation for their last consultation with the traditional healer; the above list represented the 20 most frequent problems. Other problems in the larger list included feminine sterility, paralysis, abortion, rheumatism, asthma, malaria, and bronchitis.

Supernatural problems, such as **mauvais vent** and disturbances caused by the **pangools,** represent the largest single category of problems sending a villager to a traditional healer. These supernatural problems can hardly be distinguished from mental illness and thus are most appropriately called "psycho-spiritual" problems (see **51. Etiology—Spiritual).**

93. **Treatments Received from the Healers:** Two hundred sixty-three (263) or 70.1% of **375** respondents reported that they received medicinal plants as the first line of therapy, 40 or 10.7% reported that they received baths, 24 or 6.4% reported that they received massage, and 23 or 6.1% reported that incantations were employed as the first line of therapy. As the second line of therapy, 111 of **294** or 37.8% respondents received special meals and beverages, 64 or 21.8% received baths, 44 or 15% received massage, 34 or 11.6% took in inhalations, 20 or 6.8% had incantations said over them, and 15 or 5.1% were given **gris-gris** (protective amulets).

As the third line of therapy, 42 or 38.2% of **110** respondents partook of special meals/beverages, 31 or 28.2% took in inhalations, and 16 or 14.5% were given massages.

94. **Results of Healers' Treatments (340):** Two hundred twenty (220) or 64.7% of the respondents reported that the treatment(s) given them by the healers on their last visit resulted in a complete cure. Eighty-six (86) or 25.3% of the respondents reported that their condition improved. Twenty-eight (28) or 8.2% reported that there was no change in their condition and 6 or 1.2% reported that their condition became worse after their visit to the healer. These figures indicate that

90% of the villagers in this cohort (among the valid questionnaires for this item) experienced a favorable outcome. By any measure this is a remarkable statistic. It means that, generally, for the problems that the indigenous people consult the traditional healers, these healers are successful. It might be wondered, then, why, if the healers are so accomplished, do indigenous people have such poor overall health. Simply put, health is only partly related to the existence of curative modalities; adequate, year-round nutrition, preventive health maintenance (immunizations, etc.), sanitation, and clean water are as important as curative modalities. These infrastructural obstacles to good health have not yet been surmounted in Senegal or anywhere in Africa.

95. Course of Action Taken by Patients for Conditions That Became Worse Or Did Not Improve: This item cannot be properly assessed. In the responses indicated in item no. **94,** there were just 34 patients who indicated that their condition either became worse or showed no improvement after consulting a traditional healer. Yet in this item, relating to the action taken by patients who became worse or did not improve, there are 50 valid cases (where 34 would be expected). This discrepancy cannot as yet be explained so this item cannot be analyzed or evaluated. **96. Previous Consultation with Another Traditional Healer for the Same**

Complaint (417): Three hundred forty-three (343) or 82.3% of these respondents did not previously consult a traditional healer for the problem that sent them to their last consultation with their traditional healer (no. **94),** whereas 74 or 17.7% did consult another healer prior to their last consultation. Seventy-one (71) or 98.6% of **72** of those who did consult a previous healer did follow the treatment prescribed whereas only one or 1.4% did not.

96. Previous Consultation with a Modern Practitioner (or Health Worker) for the Same Complaint (417): Two hundred fifty-six (256) or 61.4% of these respondents did not consult a modern practitioner for the same problem prior to their last consultation with their traditional healer, whereas 161 or 38.6% did previously consult a modern practitioner. Of these, 160 or 99.4% of 161 did follow the prescribed treatment.

97. Method of Payment for the Last Consultation With The Traditional Healer (414): Three hundred forty-three or 82.9% of the respondents reported paying the healer in cash, 8 or 1.9% reported paying in-kind, 4 or 1% reported paying a combination of in-kind plus cash, 57 or 13.8% reported paying nothing, and 2 or 0.5% reported that they were awaiting the outcome of treatment before making the payment.

98. Willingness to Recommend Some One to a Healer (463): Three hundred forty-six (346) or 74.7% of the respondents reported that they would recommend an acquaintance to the traditional healer, 79 or 17.1% reported that they would not, and 38 or 8.2% did not know whether they would or not.

99. Primary Problem for Which at Least 5% of the Village Respondents Indicated They Would Recommend Consultation with the Healer (270):

Problems	No. of Villagers	Valid Percentage
Mystical Disorders **(Pangools)**	71	26.3%
Mauvais Vent	26	**9.6%**
Headache & Dizzyness	26	9.6%
Divination	26	9.6%
Purification	19	7.0%
Stomachache	13	4.8%

There were 32 other primary problems listed for which the village respondents indicated they would recommend a traditional healer to some one else. The psycho-spiritual problems, as seen in the above list, clearly dominate as the motive for recommending others to a traditional healer.

100. **Has the Village Respondent Already Taken Some One to Consult the Healer (458):** Three hundred twenty-nine (329) or 71.8% of the respondents reported that they already had taken some one to the healer whereas 129 or 28.2% denied it.

101. **Relationship to the Village Respondent of the Person Taken to the Healer (328):** One hundred fifty-nine (159) or 48.5% of the respondents reported that the person taken to the healer was a son, 72 or 22% reported that the person was a daughter, 18 or 5.5% reported that the person was a wife, and 17 or 5.2% percent reported that the person was a friend. Smaller percentages of respondents reported that the person was a father, brother, sister, cousin, or niece. A very much smaller percentage reported that the person taken was a mother.

102. The Actual Condition for Which at Least 5% of the Village Respondents Took Some One to the Healer on the Last Occasion (316):

Problem	Number of Villagers	Valid Percentage
Mauvais Vent	44	13.9%
Fever	33	10.4%
Headache & Dizzyness	28	8.9%
Stomachache	18	5.7%
Mystic Illness **(Pangools)**	16	5.1%

There were 50 other conditions indicated by the village respondents that prompted them to actually take some one to the traditional healer.

103. Treatment Employed by the Healer on the Person Brought by the Village Respondent (304): Two hundred (200) or 65.8% of the respondents reported that (medicinal) plants were used by the healer, 36 or 11.8% reported that incantations were employed, 32 or 10.5% reported that special baths were prescribed, and 19 or 6.3% reported that massage was employed. Second-line therapy tended to rely on special foods/beverages, baths, inhalations, massages, and inhalations. Third-line therapy was characterized mostly by inhalation therapy, special foods/beverages, massage, and the use of **gris-gris** (amulets).

104. Outcome of Treatment by Healer on Person Brought by a Village Respondent (317): Two hundred twenty (220) or 69.4% of the respondents reported that the person they brought to the healer was cured, 49 or 15.5% reported that the person showed noticeable improvement, 18 or 5.7%

reported there was no change in the condition of the person brought to the healer, 11 or 3.5% reported that the patient became worse, and 19 or 6% reported that they didn't know the outcome. These results, showing a cure/improvement rate of 85% for persons brought to the healers by the respondents, are consistent with those in item no. **94** showing a cure/improvement rate of 90% among the respondents themselves. In fact, the slightly lower figure in this item may be related to the numbers of respondents who did not know the outcome, 19 versus 0 in item no. **94.** Thus, by the testimony of the healers' clientele, they are rendering their services with outstanding success.

N. *Utilization of Modern Medical Practitioners*

There are fewer than 500 physicians in all of Senegal to serve a population of seven million. This means that in the rural areas, the populace relies on village health workers, nurses, and midwives to provide modern primary care.

105. Consultation of Modern Practitioners (491): Four hundred sixty-four (464) or 94.5% of the respondents have consulted a modern practitioner for a health problem and just 27 or 5.5% have not. This consultation percentage of 94.5% for modern practitioners shows that they are somewhat more frequently consulted than the healers (86.4% in no. **90).**

Three hundred eighty-six (386) or 83.2% of **464** have received their modern care at a dispensary, 35 or 7.5% have received their care at a regional medical center, and 32 or 6.9% at a hospital (in Kaolack or Dakar).

106. Problems for Which at Least 10 of the Respondents Have Consulted a Modern Practitioner (459):

Problem	Number of Respondents	Valid Percentage
Stomach Disorder	49	10.7%
Headache & Dizzyness	39	8.5%
Malaria	36	7.8%
Aches & Pains	33	7.2%
Labor & Delivery	29	6.3%
Pre-natal Care	18	3.9%
Dermatosis (Skin Rash)	17	3.7%
Fever	15	3.3%
Open Wounds & Sores	13	2.8%
Vaccination	12	2.6%
Blood Pressure	12	2.6%
Kidney Disorders	10	2.2%
Diarrhea	10	2.2%

There are 52 other conditions that the respondents reported seeing a modern health practitioner for. Only 10 of the respondents reported consulting the modern practitioners for any of the psycho-spiritual disorders familiar to that populace.

107. Treatments Given by Modern Health Practitioners on the Last Visit (462): Four hundred twenty (420) or 90.9% of the respondents reported receiving medication directly for the presenting problem, 16 or 3.5% reported receiving a medication prescription, 10 or 2.2% reported receiving counseling, and 7 or 1.5% reported having surgery done. Other treatments included ointments, bandages, and massage.

For second-line therapy **(33)**, 17 reported having surgery performed.

108. **Outcome of Consultation with the Modern Health Practitioner (426):** Two hundred fifty-five or 59.9% of the respondents reported a cure of their condition, 81 or 19% reported noticeable improvement, 75 or 17.6% reported no change in their condition, and 15 or 3.5% reported a worsening of the problem. What is somewhat astonishing about these figures is that the report of a favorable outcome is noticeably less than that with the healers (78.9% vs. 90%). This can probably be explained by the under-developed medical system in the country. Rural patients rarely see a doctor even when they do come to a modern facility, medicines are in short supply, prescriptions are expensive, hospital beds are insufficient, and follow-up is erratic. Moreover, the typical villager has little confidence that modern medicine can be of help when it comes to psycho-spiritual conditions, which figure very prominently as health issues in this setting.

There is in fact readier access to the traditional healer, of which there are close to 400 in the region, than the modern practitioner. The traditional healer has, in effect, been providing primary care to these people for many centuries. The traditional medical "infrastructure" might thus be more effective in some ways than the modern medical one. Thus, the most reasonable explanation of the discrepancy of outcome between modern and traditional systems is a logistical/infrastructural one.

109. Method of Payment to the Modern Practitioner (460): Four hundred thirty-one or 93.7% or the respondents reported paying cash and 29 or 6.3% reported not paying anything.

O. *Relations Between Traditional and Modern Medicine*

110. Referred to a Modern Health Facility by the Traditional Healer (491): Seventeen (17) of the respondents reported being referred to a modern health facility by the traditional healer; 473 or 96.3% denied it. The conditions of these patients referred to the modern practitioner included: headache/dizzyness (3), stomachache (3), epilepsy (1), eye disease (1), side ache (1), asthma (1), dysmenorrhea (1), wound/open sore (1), diarrhea (1), testicular enlargment (1), chronic cough (1), aches/pains (1).

111. Referred to a Traditional Healer by a Modern Health Practitioner (490): Just seven (7) or 1.4% of the respondents reported being referred to a traditional healer by a modern health practitioner; 483 or 98.6% denied it. The conditions of these patients referred to the healer included: skin rash (1), **mauvais vent** (2), stomachache (1), parasitosis, and tumor (1).

112. Are There Diseases Not Treatable by the Traditional Healer? (491): Two hundred seventy-one (271) or 55.2% of the respondents reported that there were diseases untreatable by traditional medicine, 36 or 7.3% denied that there were diseases untreatable by traditional medicine, and 184 or 37.5% had no opinion.

113. Are There Diseases Not Treatable by Modern Medicine? (490): Three hundred sixty-nine (369) or 75.3% of the respondents reported that there were diseases untreatable by modern medicine, just 9 or 1.8% denied that there were diseases untreatable by modern medicine, and 112 or 22.9% expressed no opinion.

114. Five Most Common Illnesses Listed by Villagers as Untreatable by Traditional Healers (212):

Illnesses	Number of Respondents	Valid Percentage
Surgical Conditions	43	24.0%
Open Wounds/Sores	29	23.7%
Hernias	17	8.0%
Malaria	16	7.5%
Skin Rashes	10	4.7%

115. Five Most Common Illnesses Listed by Villagers as Untreatable by Modern Medicine (359):

Illnesses	Number of Respondents	Valid Percentage
Mystico-Spiritual Illness (**Pangools**)	121	33.7%
Mauvais Vent	102	28.4%
"Soul-eating"	41	11.4%
Seytane (Satan)	16	4.5%
Side Pain	13	3.6%

As noted above (item no. **109**), psycho-spiritual illnesses figure very prominently as health issues in this population. As these data show, the villagers have scant confidence that the remedies and therapies of modern medicine are effective against such problems. Like psychospiritual illness around the world, there are cultural specificities that define these disorders and their cure that are proof against modern medicine which sees itself (erroneously) as culture-neutral.

116. **Separation of Traditional and Modern Medicine (491):** Three hundred seventy-six (376) or 76.6% of the respondents indicated that the two systems were separate, 61 or 12.4% indicated that they were not separate, i.e., that they were comparable, 46 or 9.4% did not know, and 8 or 1.6% were of two minds on the subject (alike in some ways, different in others).

117. **Reasons for Separation (367):** Three hundred twenty-six (326) or 88.8% of the respondents indicated that the methods of the two systems were different, 9 or 2.5% indicated that the "specialties" of the two systems were different, 10 or 2.7% indicated that the underlying (philosophical) conceptions and beliefs were different, and 6 or 1.6% indicated that the knowledge of the practitioners in the two systems was different.

118. **Reasons for Comparability (61):** Forty (40) or 65.6% of the respondents indicated that the two systems had the same objective, 9 or 14.8% indicated that the two systems were complimentary, 6 or 9.8% indicated that modern medicine could be consulted if traditional medicine failed, 5 or 8.2 % indicated that both systems utilized plants, and 1 or 1.6% indicated that both systems worked for good.

119. **Should Traditional Medicine Be Preserved? (491):** Four hundred sixty (460) or 93.7% of the respondents indicated that traditional medicine should be preserved and main-

tained, 5 or 1% indicated that it shouldn't, and 26 or 5.3% expressed no opinion. As this and other data in this study show, the level of acceptance and confidence in traditional medicine in rural populace of Fatick is extraordinarily high.

120. **Attitudes Toward Officially Institutionalizing Training in Traditional Medicine (491):** Four hundred thirty-three (433) or 88.2% of the respondents agree that traditional medicine should have official standing and taught under official sponsorship, 18 or 3.7% deny that it should be, and 40 or 8.1% expressed no opinion.

IV. Comment

This present "double-survey" must be unique, or nearly so, in the study of African traditional medicine and its clientele for its size and comprehensiveness. It has represented an unprecedented opportunity to assess quantitatively the impact of the healers on their culture and society and to determine with hard numbers whether the healers still have a function to serve. Very clearly they do; the villagers' survey is a resounding vote of confidence in their favor.

Much has been said and written about traditional medicine in Senegal and in Africa but the conclusions about its efficacy, acceptability, and accessability have been largely inferential from both the **pro** and the **con** positions. Nonetheless, in recent decades, an increasing number of observers have suggested that traditional medicine is a crucial element in the solution of Africa's health problems and that it is no longer constructive to ignore or belittle it. Moreover, contrary to the sentiment prevailing a generation ago in Africa, traditional medicine shows every indication of maintaining its place for a long time and holding its own with modern medicine. Our numbers confirm these impressions unmistakably in Fatick and it is probably not too much to infer that the conclusions to be drawn from them are applicable on a broader continental scale. It might even be the case that development organizations working in Africa will find it increasingly efficacious to take the traditional healer into account where health issues are concerned.

Ostensibly, the simplest means of incorporating the traditional healer into health programs is to recruit them as "change agents" for certain practices and behaviors. Through the traditional healer, for example, one might be able to convince a local population to desist from applying cow dung to the cords of newborn infants, lessening the incidence of neo-natal tetanus. One could perhaps disseminate certain kinds of family planning messages through the traditional healer; even AIDS risk-reduction behaviors might be more effectively encouraged through the traditional healer. A few simple interventions designed to improve sanitary practices could be devised. There are any number of strategies such as this, relatively simple to impart, that could be implemented by the healers.

There are several caveats. One is that we should refrain from seeing the healers simply and solely as adjuncts and ancillaries to modern medicine, another kind of paraprofessional, as it were. Such an attitude would rightly be perceived as condescension and would ultimately be resisted by these persons who are proud of their skills and are heirs to traditions themselves centuries, even millenia, old. We will fare infinitely better with the traditional healer if we treat him/her as a colleague, showing respect and courtesy as is due.

Another consideration is that modern health care practitioners, exponents, and funders need to think about what the healer might be able to contribute to our knowledge, attitudes, and practices. Clearly, there is much we do not understand about a process as complex and multifaceted as healing that the healers do. By far and away, they excel modern medicine in "psychiatry," i.e., in the treatment of pyscho-spiritual disorders. Moreover, their knowledge of medicinal plants is impressive and we need to pay closer and more respectful attention to what they can accomplish with their herbal pharmacopeia.

What all this seems to signal is that traditional and modern health care practitioners need to begin a series of dialogues on potential areas of interface. This is undoubtedly delicate business. Most of the healers think that the underlying philosophical and practical differences between the two systems makes an amalgamation impossible and unadvisable. Most modern practitioners are no more sanguine about the prospects. But helping the unhealthy achieve good health—physical, psychological, and spiritual—is the common ingredient to both systems and a significant minority of practitioners from both systems feel that this shared **raison d'etre** is enough of a justification for dialogue to begin across the disciplines.

The evidence from the healers' survey leads us to believe that they are not ill-disposed toward modern medicine or its practitioners as such. Indeed, we know as a matter of fact that one of the reasons that our team received such a high level of co-operation (98% participation) from the healers is that they are eager for recognition from the modern health care sector. It took 4 ½ years of "ground work" before we could successfully launch this study; we need to be equally patient and painstaking about establishing a fruitful dialogue between traditional and modern medicine.

Ultimately, the healers would like to be incorporated into the national health care system, initially as a "parallel track," working synergistically with modern medicine to achieve health care for all Senegalese. Before that happens, however, several steps will have to be climbed. While there is vast room for continuing research among them, it is probably more important in the short term to think of a collaborative program, developing—in concert with the healers themselves-a project to achieve a specific, measurable health goal. Successfully completed, such a project would be the next step toward the progressive validation of the healers, leading, it is to be hoped, to incorporation into the national health system.

As has been intimated in an earlier paragraph, there are several domains that might be suitable for a traditional-modern collaboration. But it is imperative not to foreordain this, "from above," as it were. A lot of good will and mutual confidence has been generated by this study and this good faith needs to be nurtured carefully and built upon with all principals participating. We need now to meet with the healers with a few concrete ideas, listen to theirs, and collectively arrive at a viable proposal for a specific task. In a way it is potentially a "new" model of development, yet drawing on something very old—human co-operation, based on equal respect for the traditional and the modern. Respectfully submitted,

Charles S. Finch III, M.D., Principal Investigator
Atlanta, Georgia
December 3, 1992

Appendix I: Glossary of Special Terms

Pangools: The ancestral and cosmic spirits of the Serer who, in effect, control the Serer universe. A major cause of mental and/or physical illnesses is offending a **pangool.** This concept is pervasive throughout West Africa and the **pangools** are essentially the same as the **rabs** of the Lebu, the **nommo** of the Dogon, the **vodun** of the Fon, and the **orishas** of the Yoruba.

Djinn: A **djinn** is a Muslim elemental spirit, usually, though not always, of a mischievous character.

Louloup: A special category of ritual healer who is adept at performing a **lup** ceremony. This is exactly the same as an **ndepp** ceremony among the Lebu and it involves music, drumming, dances, rituals, and sacrifices designed either to placate the **pangools** or to invoke their power to achieve healing.

Saltigue: This class of Serer ritualists are primarily involved in divination. A **saltigue guerisseur** is consulted, for example, to divine the cause of illness. But **saltigues** have a larger function to fulfill: every year in the summer, they all gather at a great festival to predict the course of the coming year for the Serer community, particularly whether the rains will fall and how much. This is, of course, a matter of life and death among a farming people such as the Serer.

Yaal Pangool: These are the traditional Serer priests, those who maintain and perform the rites and ceremonies paying homage to and propitiating the **pangools.** In the past, they exerted considerable political as well as spiritual power. Even today, they command immense respect and reverence. Some of them combine within themselves functions of divination and ritual healing so that the demarcation among the **yaal pangools, louloups,** and **saltigues** is not always clear-cut. But the **yaal pangool** seems to be the highest level of priesthood.

Mauvais Vent: This is best translated as "ill wind," and is a common etiological category among the Serer. Like all traditional Africans, the Serer recognize a category of spirits that can cause no end of trouble to human beings. Mostly, these are the spirits of deceased sorcerers, witches, and others who caused evil and mischief during their lifetimes. These spirits cannot "cross the water," cannot achieve ancestorhood so they wander disembodied, continuing to cause problems for the living. Their presence, like that of any spirit, is signified by a "wind" and since they are malevolent, it is an "ill wind" or **mauvais vent** that they represent. All manner of physical and psychological disorders are attributed to **mauvais vent** by the Serer.

Seytane: This is the Serer rendering of the word for **Satan,** a concept reflecting Muslim influence. **Satan,** of course, is the Prince of Evil and anything evil that befalls a human being can thus be attributed to **seytane.**

Naques: A **naque** is a sorcerer/witch who uses his/her knowledge to bring misfortune on a person or his family. Usually, a **naque** only acts upon the request (and payment) of an enemy of the victim. Anthropologists see sorcerers and witches as sociopathic individuals within the traditional setting. Whatever the case, they are profoundly feared and loathed. Deceased **naques** can be the source of **mauvais vent.**

Anthropophagie: This term can be misunderstood since if translated literally into English as "man-eating," it connotes cannibalism. But **anthropophagie** is more properly defined as "soul-eating." **Naques,** for example, can augment their own power by siphoning off the soul power of another person, e.g., "soul-eating." Thus, not infrequently, obtundation and death of a person from unknown causes will be attributed to **anthropophagie** or soul-eating. The body of the victim remains untouched and unmarked.

These concepts seem alien to a Western mind-set but are nonetheless very real to the Serer and indigenous people all over the continent. Since these ideas are, to a large extent, culture-bound, only adepts completely versed in the culture and its rituals are in a position to manage illness brought on by these forces. Though these etiological concepts are culturally-specific, we still find that many of the objective signs and symptoms of these psycho-spiritual disorders are identical to those of well-known categories of mental illness in modern medicine. Even so, modern psychiatry has found itself only partially effective among indigenous peoples for these kind of problems, seldom achieving complete cures. The psycho-pharmacology of modern medicine is too often merely palliative whereas the traditional healer frequently has a cure rate approaching 70%.

The modern psychotherapeutic practitioner usually finds it difficult to understand how the traditional healer achieves his results. All we know is that he (and she) does.

APPENDIX II

The Oath of Sunu

Charles S. Finch, M.D.

Morehouse School of Medicine

April 30, 1985

THE OATH OF SUNU

By the great physician Iu-em-hept,[2] who is "he-who-comes-in-peace" and the father of us all who follow the Way of the Physician, I take this oath:

Verily, as God the Father[3] comes forth as the Sun, the Golden Hawk, from the ancient city of his birth[4] on the eastern banks of the Great River,[5] spreading forth his healing rays of light; verily, as God the Mother[6] comes forth as the moon, the Great Cow, the nurse of the World, her rays the milk of life; I, Sunu, the Physician, will walk the straight path, ever the servant of the Way of Truth[7] whose feather is the balance of our hearts.[8] I will consecrate myself to protect the sufferer from the nemeses of physical disease, mental suffering, and oppression of the spirit. I will hearken to the teachings of the learned ones who have shown me the Way of the Healing Art. So as God does love the sufferer so shall I love the sufferer; so as God does quicken those who walk in the Way of Truth so shall I endeavor to quicken those who pine from the afflictions of sickness.

May God the Mother keep me well and help me heal others as she did heal her Divine Son.[9] May God the Father manifest himself in the Way of Growth and Renewal. May I shun the doings of the Children of Revolt[11] who foster famine, pestilence, and affliction.

Here follow the Twelve Testaments[12] of the Physician: LIFE! STRENGTH! HEALTH![13]

1. *I will not do harm.*
2. *I will not spare myself to alleviate pain.*
3. *I will not defraud the sufferer.*
4. *I will not suffer myself uncleanliness of the body or spirit.*
5. *I will not mock the blind.*
6. *I will not injure the lame.*
7. *I will not sneer at the helpless of mind.*
8. *I will not profane the knowledge of the 'House of Life.'*[14]
9. *I will not defile the healing balm.*
10. *I will not cease to make light the burden of the dying.*
11. *I will not refuse ministrations to the poor.*
12. *I will not stir up strife between myself and my fellow physicians.*

The Way of Sunu is the Way of the Ancients, and as I tread on the Path of the Ancestors, I will endeavor to keep their spirit strong and not shame their memory. My life will not be other than the embodiment of the Way of Sunu: my life will be a beacon to all who come after me.

LIFE! STRENGTH! HEALTH!

COMMENTARY ON THE OATH OF SUNU

The Oath of Sunu was drafted at the specific request of Dr. Mwalimu Imara, Director of the Human Values in Medicine at the Morehouse School of Medicine, who rightly perceived that medical students of African decent should be able to reach back into their antiquity and pull forth something that will tie them to the ever-living stream of their history and inspire them as physicians. One of the most coherent and unified bodies of medical tradition existed in the ancient land of Kemit, "the Black Land," who recorded history and became the fountainhead of medical science. Homer testified to the unchallenged pre-eminence of Egypt in this domain when in the *Odyssey* he asserted that "in medicine, Egypt leaves the rest of the world behind." Hippocrates and Galen are just two of the more renowned physicians that adhered to a high code of ethics and evinced a deep compassion for those who suffered from all forms of illness—physical, mental, and spiritual.

The Oath of Sunu, as constructed here, takes its inspiration from the words, ideas, and practices of these practitioners of the healing art of ancient Egypt. While there never has been discovered an Oath of Sunu as such, the sentiments and ideals contained in the one created here resound through the medical and non-medical inscriptions of ancient Egypt. What has been attempted is to construct an oath that captures, as much as possible, the style of language, the tone, and the spirit of these ancient African physicians to help give meaning and purpose to African physicians in the modern age. This being said, it was also hoped that there would be something in the Oath which would touch something universal in the physician.

As part of this commentary, it was deemed necessary to explain some of the references for the edification of those not conversant with Egyptology. There was an attempt to inculcate into the Oath a tone and a style that was a blend of archaic and modern as a way of emphasizing the essential unity of past and present. Thus the "archaicisms" in the Oath, though toned down, were deliberate and necessary if the past is to inform and inspire the present. Each item in the Oath which needs further comment has been numbered item.

1. The word "sunu" is the Egyptian word for "the physician." The word "sunu" is sometimes rendered as "swenwe."

2. Iu-em-hept, sometimes called Imhotep, was, in the words of Sir William Osler, "the first figure of the physician to stand out clearly from the mists of antiquity." He was the prime minister of the Pharoah Djoser and designed the earliest of the pyramids, the so-called stepped pyramid of Saqqare. He was also known as an aphorist, but above all, he was a divinely-gifted physician whose renown was so great that he was defied as a god of medicine by the Egyptians after his death. In this form, he was also worshipped

by the Greeks some 2,500 years later in the person of the god Asclepios.

3. God the Father in this context is Ra, the Egyptian god of the sun, who by virtue of his pre-eminent position in the early Egyptian pantheon was considered the source of life.
4. The "city of the sun" was Annu, which the Greeks called Heliopolis, and mythologically it was considered the "birthplace" of the sun."
5. The "Great River" was the Nile, which the Egyptians called "Hapi." Herodotus rightly said that "Egypt is the gift of the river" and its waters were thought to have life-giving and healing properties.
6. God the mother in this context is Isis who is also identified with Hathor. Both Goddesses had the title "Mother of Gods," both were identified with the moon, and both had the cow as their symbol. Isis, in particular, was indispensable in the healing rituals because only she had the power to drive poison and sickness away.
7. The "Way Of Truth" was personified in the goddess Maat by the Egyptians. Her symbol was the feather and it was through her that right, truth, justice, and order reigned.
8. In the ritual for the dead, called "the Coming Forth by Day," the deceased is presented to Osiris, the Great Judge, and his heart, which contains the sum total of his thoughts, words, and deeds, is weighed on the "scale of justice." The balance on the opposite scale is the "feather of Truth (Maat)" and in order to attain salvation, the heart could not outweigh the feather.

9. The "Divine Son" is Horus, a figure of the newborn sun; also of the youthful solar hero-god who slays the dragon of darkness. As an infant, Horus is stung by a scorpion and is only saved by the timely intervention of his mother Isis.
10. In Egypt, God as a personification of Growth and Renewal was Osiris who as the god of resurrection signifies the conquest of sickness and death.
11. The "Children of Revolt" are the followers of Apep, the Evil One. They are those who bring every kind of calamity into the world.
12. The "Twelve Testaments" were inspired by the so-called "42 Negative Confessions" which are contained in the *Egyptian Book of the Dead*, more properly called the *Book of the Coming Forth By Day.* These Negative Confessions are also the prototypes of the Biblical Ten Commandments.
13. These three words were always pronounced whenever the name of the Pharoah was mentioned. In the context here, they seemed particularly suitable.
14. The "House of Life," or "Per Ankh," is where Egyptian physicians and savants studied. There was usually one associated with every major temple and each contained a library, a hospital, a musical conservatory and all the other accouterments of a full-fledged university.

The numerous Greek savants, including Pythagorus, Thales, and Plato who were known to have undertaken their formal education in Egypt, studied in these Houses of Life.

It is hoped that this Commentary has shed some light on the various references in the Oath thus making it more comprehensible to all. The day may yet come when all of this will be a part of the general fund of knowledge, thus making this Commentary unnecessary.

Charles S. Finch, M.D.
Morehouse School of Medicine
April 30, 1985

Index

B

C

D

E

F

G

H

N

O

P

Q

R

S

T

U

V

W

Y

Z